INFORMATION OVERLOAD

FRAMEWORK, TIPS, AND TOOLS TO MANAGE IN
COMPLEX HEALTHCARE ENVIRONMENTS

Mary C. Sitterding, PhD, RN, CNS and
Marion E. Broome, PhD, RN, FAAN, Editors

American Nurses Association

Silver Spring, Maryland • 2015

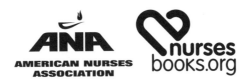

American Nurses Association
8515 Georgia Avenue, Suite 400
Silver Spring, MD 20910-3492
1-800-274-4ANA
www.NursingWorld.org

Published by Nursesbooks.org
The Publishing Program of ANA
www.Nursesbooks.org/

The American Nurses Association (ANA) is the only full-service professional organization representing the interests of the nation's 3.1 million registered nurses through its constituent/state nurses associations and its organizational affiliates. The ANA advances the nursing profession by fostering high standards of nursing practice, promoting the rights of nurses in the workplace, projecting a positive and realistic view of nursing, and by lobbying the Congress and regulatory agencies on healthcare issues affecting nurses and the public.

Library of Congress Cataloging-in-Publication Data
Information overload (Sitterding)
  Information overload: framework, tips, and tools to manage in complex healthcare environments / Mary C. Sitterding and Marion E. Broome, editors.
    p. ; cm.
  Includes bibliographical references and index.
  ISBN 978-1-55810-607-9 (pbk. : alk. paper)
  I. Sitterding, Mary C., 1960- , editor. II. Broome, Marion, editor. III. American Nurses Association, issuing body. IV. Title.
  [DNLM: 1. Nursing Care. 2. Communication. 3. Evidence-Based Nursing. 4. Health Information Management. 5. Medical Errors--prevention & control. 6. Mental Fatigue--prevention & control. WY 100.1]
  RT51
  610.73—dc23
                         2015004758

978-1-55810-607-9   SAN: 851-3481   04/2015
First printing: April 2015

Contents

Information Overload!
An Introduction

My phone rings every five minutes regardless of what I'm doing.
I might be trying to check a chart. I'm helping a patient. I'm giving
medicine. I'm talking with a student nurse, if I'm fortunate enough to
have one that I'm working with that day. It could be the unit secretary
saying, "Patient 42 wants ice." Or they need to go to the bathroom. Or
they need pain meds. Or it could be the PICC team, and it happened
to me this morning, calling me saying, "Is there any reason this patient
can't have a line in his arm?" I wasn't even in that patient's room!
How can I see what's going on? It's very difficult, to be honest. I very
nearly always answer the phone. The only times that I don't are when
the battery goes dead. The battery tends to go dead about 11:00. It's just
really hard to always know what's going on.

—Medical–surgical nurse during a typical day of overload
(Sitterding et al., 2012 p. 87)

Consider your role in this narrative. You might be this direct care nurse.
You might be this nurse's nurse manager, division director, or chief nurse.
Maybe you're an advanced practice nurse tasked to impact direct care
nurse clinical decision-making. Maybe you are the nurse educator or
faculty partner responsible for preparing the next generation of direct care
nurses, nurse leaders, and nurse educators. Maybe you provide the link
integrating research, practice, and informatics eliminating unnecessary
work for nurses. Or maybe you are the consulting architect who is asked
to design space that will "eliminate unnecessary information". Information
or cognitive overload is an interpretation a nurse makes in response to
breakdowns or imbalances between cognitive demand and capacity. The
situation-in-context, nurse expertise, and his or her ability to make sense
and act upon the situation in context determine the interpretation of overload. In this book, we strive to bring the readers to a better understanding
of the numerous factors that influence each nurse's interpretation of the
information and cues that she/he are dealing with every day in practice.

Information is critical for the nurse to provide the highest quality, safest care possible. Consumer demand for safe, timely, effective, efficient, equitable, and patient-centric care is here to stay. Value-based care and risk-based payment structures are here to stay. The demand for highly reliable, safe patient care is here to stay. It's your role and your response to these demands that is alterable. We believe the imperative to address the economic and human burden of health care is urgent and very real. We believe that in this book our interprofessional colleagues bring a framework, tips, and tools to address—at least in part—some of the issues contributing to information overload in nursing. We have much to learn but the evidence, perspectives, and experiences of the authors of this book lay a solid foundation of knowledge on which to build.

About This Book

The purpose of this book is to provide you with a framework to think about information overload and the various factors and contexts that influence its effect on care providers and thus the patient and family. We also provide case exemplars to help you apply the framework and knowledge in the text, as well as tips and tools that might be helpful references as you interpret and embrace the opportunity to alter your interpretation of overload. The material covered is relevant to all levels of nurses practicing in healthcare organizations and academic institutions, and is structured such that you can weave in and out of chapters relevant to your particular area of interest and situation-in-context.

Chapter 1, *An Overview of Information Overload,* introduces you to the idea of information overload and factors within your current work environment that might be influencing your interpretation of information overload. At the completion of Chapter 1, you will have a basic understanding and be compelled to learn more about this phenomenon influencing nursing and patient care safety.

Chapter 2, *Information Overload: A Framework for Explaining the Issues and Creating Solutions,* provides a framework that explains the cognitive work of the individual nurse. Relationships between clinical decision-making in transition and proposed factors influencing work complexity contributors. Knowledge in context, situation awareness, management of competing goals, cognitive stacking, and clinical judgments influencing nursing practice, patient, nursing, and system outcomes are described and illustrative examples provided. At the completion of Chapter 2, you will have a framework to consider—in part—those factors influencing the interpretation of overload as it relates to the individual cognitive work of the nurse.

Chapter 3, *Information Architecture*, provides the perspective of information and organizational architecture, and considerations to counter the complexity within workspace and workflow design. At the completion of Chapter 3, you will have practical tactics enabling you to assess and mitigate workflow and workspace barriers influencing non-value added nurse work contributing to information overload.

Chapter 4, *Leadership in a Complex World*, provides the perspective of the nurse leader who must embrace the opportunity to alter the interpretation of overload, leveraging the energy and creative genius on the edge of complexity. At the completion of Chapter 4, you will walk away with tools to unlock your and your team's unlimited potential for adaptation, resilience, and agility.

Chapter 5, *The Clinical Nurse Specialists (CNSs) as Change Agents*, introduces you to the perspective of the change agent clinical nurse specialist and, through an exemplar, provides tips and tools to mitigate overload and positively influence change acceleration in an organization.

Chapter 6, *Supporting Leaders Through Complexity and Information Overload*, provides reflections and wisdom on leadership from an experienced healthcare system nurse executive. Using an interview format, it reveals leadership as an emotional state grounded in core values and how leadership competencies are essential to lead and manage in a volatile, uncertain, chaotic, and ambiguous world.

About the Authors

Mary C. Sitterding, PhD, RN, CNS, serves as Executive Director, Nursing Research, Professional Practice, and Operational Improvement at Indiana University Health in Indianapolis, Indiana. Dr. Sitterding received her doctorate at the Indiana University School of Nursing. Dr. Sitterding is recognized for her research in individual nursing situation awareness and safety organizing. She is published in top-tier research journals including the Western Journal for Nursing Research and Medical Care. Additional areas of expertise include the examination of the cognitive and relational mechanisms influencing nursing work and patient care safety. She has presented nationally and is recognized for her expertise in patient safety, quality, complex adaptive systems, change management, diffusion of innovation, and professional nursing practice. Dr. Sitterding has served as a peer reviewer for a number of journals and also serving as guest editor for publications on patient safety. Dr. Sitterding is a member of the American Nurses Association, Sigma Theta Tau International, and American Organization of Nurse Executives (AONE). Dr. Sitterding has served on the AONE Patient Safety and Quality Committee and currently serves the AONE Nursing Research Committee. Dr. Sitterding also serves as an Appraiser for the Magnet Recognition Program, American Nurses Credentialing Center.

Marion E. Broome, PhD, RN, FAAN, was appointed Dean and Professor, Vice-Chancellor for Nursing Affairs at Duke University, and Associate Vice-President for Academic Affairs at Duke University Health System in Durham, NC. Prior to this, she was University Dean and Distinguished Professor at Indiana University School of Nursing and Associate Vice-President of Academic Affairs at Indiana University Health 2004–2014. Dr. Broome has held faculty positions in schools of nursing at the Medical College of Georgia and Rush University in Chicago, IL; held an endowed chair in pediatrics at the Children's Hospital of Wisconsin and the University of Wisconsin at Milwaukee; and was associate dean for research at the University of Alabama at Birmingham School of Nursing. As a pre-eminent scholar in the healthcare field, she has published over 100 articles in refereed journals in a variety of disciplines, 10 chapters, and 5 books. She is currently editor-in-chief of *Nursing Outlook*, the official journal of the American Academy of Nursing and the Council for the Advancement of Nursing Science. Dr. Broome consults with a variety of schools of nursing and Magnet designated hospitals related to evidence-based practice programs, research implementation, and professional development programs for nurses and faculty.

Patricia Ebright, PhD, RN, CNS, has healthcare experience that includes 42 years as a registered nurse, with the first 28 years as staff nurse, nurse manager, and clinical nurse specialist in acute care hospital settings. Since completing a nursing doctorate in 1998 at Indiana University, she has been teaching in undergraduate and graduate nursing programs. Her research focus is on work complexity for healthcare providers and the link between complexity and care delivery systems, implementation of change in systems, and patient safety. She was a member of the first Patient Safety Leadership Fellowship class sponsored by the National Patient Safety Foundation and currently collaborates with IU Health, Indianapolis, on patient safety/quality programs.

Tim Tarnowski, MBA, MIM, is Senior Vice President and Chief Information Officer at UMass Memorial Health Care. Tim has been a healthcare IT executive for the past 25 years. Prior to joining UMass in November 2014, he served in executive IT leadership roles at IU Health, University of Kentucky Healthcare, and at Stanford Hospitals and Clinics. Tim has been accountable for leading transformational change initiatives, establishing IT governance models, planning and execution of IT strategies, and overall IT restructuring activities. During this time he has successfully led several large, enterprise-wide EMR and financial systems implementations. Tim serves as a Board member for LHP Software, LLC.

Terri Bogue, MSN, RN, PCNS, is a board-certified pediatric clinical nurse specialist with over 25 years of experience in pediatric nursing. Her publications and presentations focus on improving patient outcomes and reducing hospital-acquired infections. She currently practices at Riley Hospital for Children at Indiana University Health in Indianapolis, Indiana.

Robert L. Bogue, MCSE, CNA, is an international speaker and author of more than 25 books. He is a twelve-time recipient of the Microsoft Most Valuable Professional Award. In his consulting practice, Robert helps some of the world's largest organizations reach their potential.

Jason H. Gilbert, BSN, MBA, RN, is currently the Director of Nursing Operations at IU Health Methodist Hospital in Indianapolis, Indiana. He has worked in progressive leadership roles in large complex healthcare organizations nationally. His scholarly interests include leadership and change management in complex organizations. He is currently a PhD student at the Indiana University School of Nursing where he is studying the effects of intellectual capital on patient and organizational outcomes.

Linda Q. Everett, PhD, RN, FAAN, NEA-BC, is the immediate past Executive Vice President and Chief Nurse Executive at Indiana University Health (formerly Clarian Health) in Indianapolis, Indiana. In 2007, she was president of the American Organization of Nurse Executives (AONE). Previously, she was the long-time chief nursing officer at the University of Iowa Hospital and Clinics. At IU Health, Dr. Everett provided leadership to staff at Methodist Hospital, University Hospital, Riley Hospital for Children and Saxony Hospital—one of the Midwest's largest healthcare systems— and is responsible for staff across many disciplines and specialty areas of care delivery, including pharmacy, rehabilitation services, and case management. She also coordinates nursing practice and polices across the statewide IU Health system, including 18 additional hospitals; lends strategic planning and workforce development support to the IU Health executive team; and serves as associate dean for clinical affairs at the Indiana University School of Nursing. An active researcher, lecturer and speaker, Dr. Everett is widely published on nursing management and patient care topics. Among her many honors are being named a Woman of Influence in 2006 by an Iowa business journal; serving in a leadership role for AONE; being named a fellow in the American Academy of Nursing; and completing the Johnson & Johnson Wharton Fellows Program in Management for Nurse Executives at the University of Pennsylvania in Philadelphia.

Acknowledgments

I would like to acknowledge each and every clinical nurse who volunteered to participate in the conduct of research revealing the invisible cognitive work of the nurse and factors contributing to overload. Your participation in this research illuminated the economic value of the nurse and the healthcare delivery team. I would like to acknowledge my nursing leadership colleagues who applied and prioritized the cognitive work of the nurse framework each and every time a near miss or adverse event occurred. I would like to thank Dr. Marion Broome for her unwavering commitment to integrate and align research, practice, and education, recognizing her generosity of spirit leading, coaching, and mentoring. I would especially like to thank Dr. Patricia Ebright for inspiring the extension of her seminal contribution on the cognitive work of nursing framework.

—*Mary C. Sitterding*

I would like to thank my nursing colleagues (faculty, advanced practice nurses, and graduate students) I have worked with this past decade. Each in their own way and time has taught me so much about how to navigate complexities in the intersecting and interdependent worlds of academe and practice. The core values these nurses hold—integrity, sharing of self, persistence, and self-reflection—are why we, as a profession, have managed to keep our laser-focus on the well-being of patients and their families. And these shared values are what inspire me to continue to contribute to the discourse about how to lead through the chaotic waters of health care we are now navigating together.

—*Marion E. Broome*

1

An Overview of Information Overload

Mary C. Sitterding, PhD, RN, CNS

The Burning Platform

"It started out with just the noise of the baby crying—and you know that sort of sets you a little on edge. I didn't notice the IV rates. It was while we were doing all this stuff and the nurse is going to help give the flush for the phenobarb and start other IV fluids or whatever...all of a sudden the nurse standing behind me said, 'Why is his hyperalimentation going at 360 an hour?' And I said, 'It's supposed to be 36 an hour.' My stomach just went to the floor."

—RN, 2–5 years experience

The human and economic burden of information overload often experienced in the form of patient care error is well documented (Barker et al., 2011; Cohen, 2007; Institute of Medicine, 2000; Kopp et al., 2006; Sharek & Classen, 2006). Nursing work environments are emotionally exhausting, attentionally demanding, and increasingly complex (Ebright et al., 2003; Vogus et al., 2010; Sitterding et al., 2014; Vogus et al., 2014). Nursing work-related fatigue has become increasingly more prevalent with nurses reporting sleep disturbances on one-third of their work days (Smith-Miller et al., 2014). The impact of nurse fatigue on attention and information interpretation is remarkable and may produce effects of information overload illustrated in change and inattentional blindness resulting in patient care error.

What Is Information Overload?

Information or cognitive overload is defined as an interpretation that people make in response to breakdowns, interruptions of ongoing projects, or imbalances between demand and capacity (Weick, 2009, p. 76). The interpretation of an overload is affected by the situation at hand. One must make sense of interruptions and understand the types of and responses to interruptions in the context of the developmental level of the registered nurse or their level of expertise (Weick, 2009; Benner, 2009). Numerous assumptions underlie the argument that information overload is isolated to information processing:

1. Meaning representation and computation are the primary cognitive organizational activities, as opposed to construction and interpretation; cognitive organization is a finite container overfilled with demands;
2. Communication channels have fixed information limits; attention is a scarce resource; short-term storage is limited; and
3. Output must be formulated in response to input with a fixed time interval (Weick, 2009).

Weick challenges that information overload is not only an isolated problem of information processing, but is also an issue of interpretation and the inability to make sense of perceived demands, capabilities, data, and the situation at hand (Weick, 2009). Interpretation lessons are necessary for making sense of a situation and offering a mitigated information overload solution, which opposes the cognitive work of decision-making that taxes or amplifies overload.

Information Overload and Expertise

The follow quote is an excerpt from an interview with an expert nurse during a study completing a hybrid concept analysis on situation awareness in nursing (Sitterding et al., 2012). The investigators used cognitive task analysis techniques to understand the cognitive work of the direct care nurse and what factors influenced how and what the direct care nurse paid attention to in the course of the average day on an inpatient unit.

> *It's just a multitude of things. I have a list of one hundred things to do in twelve hours. Yes, that's what it feels like. And it's overwhelming. I know I miss things.*

> *I was in the Navy for 4 years. Every alarm has a certain meaning and action that you have to take. I've carried that in my practice. I place value on every sound I hear—I knew that [noise] was [the patient's] vent alarm and he was in trouble. I knew he popped his vent off.*
> —Expert Nurse

Benner and colleagues describe the expert nurse as one demonstrating embodied intelligence. Expert nurses not only know what to do and when to do it, but know how to do what is needed (Benner et al., 1999, p. 558). Essentially, how nurses use knowledge in actual situations determines expertise. Determining a nurse's level of expertise includes knowing the following: (1) what the nurse brings to the situation at hand; and (2) how the nurse cognitively organizes what they know to make inferences about the situation at hand and what they can expect to happen, and the extent to which the knowledge can be activated in that particular situation. Thus, the question is not simply whether or not the nurse has the knowledge, but whether in that situation the relevant knowledge is activated and acted upon (Benner et al., 1999; Ebright et al., 2003; Sitterding et al., 2012).

> *One of the newer nurses called for me—she noticed the rhythm was different but she didn't know what to make of it. I took a look at the rhythm. I had seen it before and knew nothing was happening with this guy's ventricles. I grabbed the code cart and started compressions.*
> —Expert Nurse

Knowledge is limited in novice and advanced beginner nurses, which means subtle cues about the patient's condition and/or work environment might be missed, leading to inattentional or change blindness. Weick (2009) defends the implication that overload is about action, interpretation, and sense-making. He asserts that when action is the central focus, interpretation—not decision-making—is the core phenomenon underscoring the importance of framing error within a culture of safety, about good nurses trying to make sense of a situation rather, than bad nurses making poor decisions.

Information Overload, Task Management, Interruptions, and Time Pressures

So, you're in the midst of care and people just call out questions to you. And you have to sort of change how you're thinking to answer, "What was the lab on that kid down the hall?" and a few minutes later a nurse comes in and says, "Can you help me out with this kid?" Or "Do you know where Doreen is who's working next to you?" "Well, uh, no, I don't know where she is." Or, a secretary comes over the intercom and says "So and so is on the phone" or they have a message for you. I mean, work-related, but still, it's those little things that happen all the time and no amount of smart pump technology gets you by any of that. You miss things."

—Nurse (<2 years' experience)

Interruptions and time pressures are related to information overload. However, time pressures and interruptions are not all bad, depending on how one interprets them. Interruptions in nursing care can disturb the flow of tasks, or even bring workflow to a halt (Weick, 2009). Additionally, interruptions can trigger feelings of time pressure, particularly in new nurse graduates. Workplace interruptions have been identified as primary factors influencing the nurse's work environment and may influence patient care error (McGillis et al., 2010; Sitterding et al., 2014). Although the majority of direct care nurses immediately engage when interrupted, the assumption that interruptions have only negative effects on nursing care is unsubstantiated and underlies the idea that it is more important to understand how the nurse makes sense of the interruption in context or in the situation at hand (Weick, 2009; Hopkinson & Jennings, 2013; Sitterding et al., 2014). The interpretation and effects of interruptions on information overload are related to working memory load, interruption similarity, interruption position, interruption modality, and expertise (Li et al., 2012).

Information Overload and Capacity

You prioritize, pretty much, by the kid who needs the most ... who's the sickest, who's got the most drips hanging ... the most labile. That's how you automatically give priority. Patient satisfaction is a big deal, but you have to prioritize so you can keep an eye on things. I was interrupted by a mom who asked for chocolate milk for her son. You decide chocolate milk versus dopamine drip for my other kid who's in greater need.

—Expert Nurse

Weick (2009) asserts that information overload is not only the result of excessive input, but may also be the result of limited capacity. Factors that negatively impact limited cognitive capacity in nursing include: increasing task demands, competing task demands, and complex task demands. Additionally, capacity is limited when time is short, when performance or production pressures are looming, and when there is too little control in terms of processing the input (Weick, 2009).

Attentional Factors Influencing the Information Capacity Tipping Point

I barely remember who I got a report from that morning, let alone the times when morning blood sugars were recorded ... it's a very busy unit with high acuity patients. We're sending patients home, we're getting patients in ... it's easy to get bogged down and miss things.

—Nurse, 2–5 year's experience

Attentional tunneling has been described as phenomena where scanning is decreased and attention is locked in on certain aspects or features of the environment. Factors influencing nurse attention are (Endsley, 2000):

1. Attentional tunneling
2. Prerequisite memory trap
3. Workload, anxiety, and other stressors
4. Data overload
5. Misplaced salience
6. Complexity creep
7. Errant mental models
8. Out-of-the-loop syndrome

The result is that nurses intentionally or inadvertently drop their scanning behavior. Successful attention is dependent on constantly juggling different aspects of the environment. The problem is not physical interference, but attentional distraction—switching attention (Endsley, 2000).

Working memory is another distinguishing factor differentiating high and low levels of attention. It is noteworthy that the literature infers a relationship between knowledge or experiential learning, working memory, and situational awareness (Endsley, 2000; Wickens, 2008). There is a consistent theme of differentiating attention awareness among experts and novices. Novices—in any industry or discipline—have limited working memory to perceive multiple sources of information, interpret, and project the future status based upon that information. Endsley refers to the fact that the memory bank is essentially limited, meaning that people can hold seven (± two) chunks of information in working or short-term memory. Scanning requires that previously accessed information can be combined with new information in a proccess referred to as chunking (Endsley, 2003). It is known that over-reliance on memory contributes to patient care error (IOM, 1999).

Stressors significantly strain nurse attention. Stress can be the result of anxiety or frustration about the nursing work in context, relationships influencing the nursing work, or the result of time pressures, mental workload, or uncertainty—all common in many healthcare environments. Endsley (2003) proposes that the negative impacts of stress on attention, specifically causing a decrease in memory absorption and retention, typically result in nurses arriving at a decision without considering all available information.

Misplaced salience and errant mental models negatively influence attention, triggering information overload. A nurse will seek information that's consistent with and contributes to their particular goals. Salience is defined as follows, "the compellingness of certain forms of information is largely determined by physical characteristics" (Endsly, 2003, p. 37). Healthcare environments have been designed to draw nurse attention to what's been defined by regulatory bodies and others as important. However, inappropriately designed and/or overused physical signals such as a flashing light or auditory alarm within the work environment can distract nurse attention from more important information, including subtle changes in the patient's condition, relevant information within the electronic health record, or high-risk medication dosage discrepancies between micrograms and milligrams.

Errant mental models negatively influence nurse attention, as these are situations where important cues are misinterpreted. The nurse retrieves the wrong mental model, leading to misinterpretation, which can result in information overload. Consider the very busy emergency room nurse in triage making decisions about where to place the child who is admitted with nausea and vomiting at camp that summer. Consider the nurse response when the less-experienced resident suggests the child is of low acuity, placing him at the bottom of the priority list. Consider the nurse's mental model and experience with these symptoms in children. Consider subtle cues requiring the nurse's attention to differentiate between benign nausea and vomiting and something a little more serious—diabetic keto-acidosis, for example.

Consider the nursing work environment. Consider the uncertainty, speed, volume, and complexity of constant and competing data input for the average registered nurse who is interrupted every three minutes and completes more than 50% of their tasks in less than 30 seconds (Cornell et al.).

The imperative to address nurse attention and information overload in health care is real. We are required to rapidly accelerate our capacity to provide better care at a lower cost. We are required to eliminate unnec- essary waste within the healthcare environment. We strive to adopt high-reliability behaviors, but have not designed care delivery environments or processes that enable high-reliability behaviors. In these settings, nurses are overwhelmed and on overload—information overload.

We seek to provide an interprofessional response to the concept of information overload within the existing healthcare environment. The response includes a framework that describes, explains, and predicts the cognitive work of the individual nurse, leadership strategies within a complex adaptive environment, tips and tools that address attention to self and attention to the system, and wisdom from a sage.

References

Aiken, L. H., Smith, H. L., & Lake, E. T. (1994). Lower Medicare mortality among a set of hospitals known for good nursing care. *Medical Care, 32*(8), 771–787.

Barker, K. N., Flynn, E. A., Pepper, G. A., Bates, D. W., & Mikeal, R. L. (2002). Medication errors observed in 36 health care facilities. *Archives of Internal Medicine, 162*(16), 1897–1903.

Benner, P., Tanner, C. A., & Chesla, C. A. 2009. *Expertise in nursing practice: Caring, clinical judgment, and ethics* (2nd ed.). New York, NY: Springer Publishing.

Benner, P. (1999). *From novice to expert: Excellence and power in clinical nursing practice.* Menlo Park, CA: Addison-Wesley.

Classen D., Resar R., Griffin F., Federico, F., Frankel, T., Kimmel, N., Whittington, J. C., Frankel, A., Seger, A., & James, B. C. (2011). Global trigger tool shows that adverse events in hospitals may be ten times greater than previously measured. *Health Affairs, 30*(4), 581–589.

Cook, R. I., & Woods, D. D. (1994). Operating at the sharp end: The complexity of human error. In Edward Boger (Ed.), *Human Error in Medicine* (225–310). Hillsdale, NJ: Lawrence Erlbaum Associates.

Cornell, P., Riordan, M., Townsend-Gervis, M., & Mobley, R. (2011). Barriers to critical thinking: Workflow interruptions and task switching among nurses. *Journal of Nursing Administration, 41*(10), 407–414.

Donabedian, A. (1980). *The definition of quality and approaches to its assessment (Explorations in Quality Assessment and Monitoring, Vol 1).* Ann Arbor, MI: Health Administration Press.

Ebright P., Urden L., Patterson E., & Chalko, B. (2004). Themes surrounding novice nurse near-miss and adverse event situations. *Journal of Nursing Administration, 34,* 11.

Endsley M. R., & Garland, D. J. (2000). *Situational awareness analysis and measurement.* Mahwah, NJ: Lawrence Erlbaum Associates.

Endsley, M. R., & Garland, D. J. (2000). "Theoretical underpinnings of situational awareness: A critical review." In M. R. Endsley & D. J. Garland (Eds.), *Situational awareness analysis and measurement* (3–32). Mahwah, NJ: Lawrence Erlbaum Associates.

Facione, Noreen C. & Facione, Peter A. (2008). Critical thinking and clinical judgment. In Noreen C. Facione & Peter A. Facione (Eds.), *Critical Thinking and Clinical Reasoning in the Health Sciences: A Teaching Anthology* (1–13). Millbrae, CA: California Academic Press.

Fonteyn, M. E., & Fisher, A. (1995). Use of think aloud method to study nurses' reasoning and decision making in clinical practice settings. *Journal of Neuroscience Nursing, 27,* 124–128.

Institute of Medicine. (2000). *To err is human: Building a safer health system.* Washington, DC: National Academy Press.

Kalisch, B., Landstrom, G., & Williams, R. (2009). Missed nursing care: Errors of omission. *Nursing Outlook, 57*(1), 3–9.

Kohn, L. T., Corrigan, J. M., & Donaldson, M. S. (Eds.). (2000). To err is human: Building a safer health system. *Committee on Quality of Health Care in America, Institute of Medicine.* Washington, DC: National Academy Press. Retrieved from http://books.nap.edu/catalog/9728.html

Kopp, B. J., Erstad, B. L., Allen, M. E., Theodorou, A. A., & Priestley, G. (2006). Medication errors and adverse drug events in an intensive care unit: Direct observation approach for detection. *Critical Care Medicine, 34,* 415–25.

Krichbaum, K., Diemert, C., Jacox, L., Jones, A., Koenig, P., Mueller, C., & Disch, J. (2007). Complexity compression: nurses under fire. *Nursing Forum, 42*(2).

Patterson, E. S., Ebright, P., & Saleem, J. (2011). Investigating stacking: How do registered nurses prioritize their activities in real time? *International Journal of Industrial Ergonomics, 41*: 389–393.

Sitterding, M., Broome, M., Everett, L., & Ebright, P. (2012). Situational awareness in nursing: A hybrid concept analysis. *Advances in Nursing Science, 35*(1), 77-92.

Sitterding, M., Ebright, P., Broome, M., Patterson, E., & Wuchner, S. (2014). Situational awareness and interruption handling during medication administration. *Western Journal Nursing Research, 36*(7), 891-916.

Tucker, A. L., & Spear, S. J. (2006). Operational failures and interruptions in hospital nursing. *Health Services Research Journal, 41*(3), 643-662.

Vogus, T., Sutcliff, K. M., & Weick, K. E. (2010). Doing no harm: Enabling, enacting, and elaborating a culture of safety in health care. *Academy of Management Perspectives, 24*, 60-77.

Vogus, T., Cooil, B., Sitterding, M., & Everett, L. (2014). Safety organizing, emotional exhaustion, and turnover in hospital nursing units. *Medical Care, 52*(10), 870-876.

Weick, K. E., & Sutcliffe, K. M. (2007). *Managing the unexpected: Resilient performance in an age of uncertainty* (2nd ed). San Francisco, CA: Jossey-Bass.

Wickens, C., McCarley, J. (2008). *Applied attention theory*. Boca Raton, FL: CRC Press.

Wickens, C. D., & Hollands, J. (2000). *Engineering psychology and human performance* (3rd ed). Upper Saddle River, NJ: Prentice Hall.

Woods, D. D., Johannesen, L. J., Cook, R. I., & Sarter, N. B. (1994). Behind human error: Cognitive systems, computers, and hindsight. Columbus, OH: Crew Systems Ergonomic Information and Analysis Center.

2

Information Overload: A Framework for Explaining the Issues and Creating Solutions

Mary C. Sitterding, PhD, RN, CNS and Patricia Ebright, PhD, RN, CNS

Case Study

The average nurse experiences a multitude of competing and continuous sources of information throughout their work shift. On any given day, a nurse is managing information about patients, unit priorities, other nurses, and team members—all at once. The vulnerability for cognitive or information overload is real. Stella—an experienced emergency department charge nurse—is an expert nurse; how she manages information or the cognitive work of nursing can be illustrated through the Cognitive Work of Nursing framework. Stella's narrative follows.

On Saturday, I was in charge and I thought to myself, I'm doing two jobs today. I'm keeping an eye on the falls work, the IOPO work, I'm in charge. I got unit committee stuff, and I'm also helping out with Constant Care. I can just tell how things are going.

I can just tell by the communication overhead how things are going and what I need to be paying attention to. You know, you can see. You can just see. The ambulance guys are walking in and out. You can hear the secretary overhead saying, "new patient coming in." You can see triage people. You can see folks walking back and forth. I can just tell when we're busy and what I need to pay attention to. I typically pick a place where I can be most helpful. How I know which place to pick, how do I know, as charge, where I need to spend my time? I look at the expressions of other nurses' faces. I can tell by looking at them. I can tell if they look overwhelmed. Or I can hear. You know, you hear an ambulance report and you know that that nurse down the hall, they're going to need an extra set of hands. So, even though I'm in the middle of taking a med into a patient's room, I might stop what I'm doing and go and help out that nurse if I feel like they're overwhelmed.

—Expert Nurse

I know what and when to expect it. I know depending on the ambulance report that I hear overhead, I know that they're going to be sick. I know that when the ambulance guys call me that they need me. That's why we have two charge nurses. I also know when Constant Care forwards their phone to me, that's when I really know that I need to stop what I'm doing and pay attention. So, even if I'm in the middle of taking a med to a patient in another room, if we're busy, we forward our calls to each other. I'll forward my calls to the Constant Care nurse and she'll forward her calls to me. So when I know when those calls start coming toward me, if the calls are forwarded to me, I know that she is overwhelmed and I know that I really need to help her out. It happens. We can make mistakes.

—Expert Nurse

Information overload happens every day on every unit in every hospital.

Understanding the Invisible Work of Nursing: The Cognitive Work of Nursing Framework

Consider the volume and rate of information at any given time for the average direct care nurse. Consider technology as just one data source. Gold and colleagues discovered great density in the average intensive care unit, with nearly 1,800 data points per patient per day. Consider other data sources described by Stella—what she heard and saw, and how she processed incoming information. Consider the number of times Stella mentioned knowing, seeing, and hearing. Consider how Stella prioritized (or stacked) her nursing work, including how she handled interruptions. Consider that Stella was concerned about her nurse coworker experiencing information overload and how she prioritized the calls forwarded to her from her nurse coworker.

Exactly what is it that supports Stella's decision-making that results in desired patient outcomes? What factors interfered with Stella's coworker's decision-making to the extent that she was on information overload and was forwarding her calls to Stella? Answering these questions requires an understanding of the complexity of the cognitive work required during actual care situations, which leads to decisions about care. In this chapter, we propose a framework to explain how the cognitive work of nursing in actual work situations is determined by contextual factors in the environment (environmental demands) that influence information processing, decision-making, and judgments about nursing care delivered in three important ways. This framework proposes the following:

1. Continuously changing environmental demands challenges the ability of the registered nurse (RN) to attend to the present situation.
2. These demands can lead to multiple and competing RN goals for care.
3. These factors inform judgments about the prioritization of care for patient safety and quality outcomes.

The Cognitive Work of Nursing Framework (CWNF) represents the complexity of RN work in actual care situations. The framework depicts relationships among the following:

1. Environmental factors (Work Complexity Contributors)
2. Cognitive work leading to decisions about care (Clinical Reasoning-in-Transition)
3. Immediate outcomes of the cognitive work (Clinical Judgments)
4. Nursing care delivered and patient, nurse, and system outcomes

We consider this framework to be in the developmental stage, with multiple opportunities for future research. The framework described here—and its future development—informs the design of healthcare environments, practice, education, and policy initiatives to support RNs in the actual work of nursing practice including information management.

Background

The proposed framework for representing the work of RNs is based on the Cognitive Work at the Sharp End of Practice framework developed in 1994 (Cook et al.). Cook, Woods, and Johansen (1994) represented what it is like to work in actual situations involving real life contexts and complexity.

For example, at the point of care delivery (i.e., sharp end), nurses are involved in constantly evolving situations. Recall Stella's narrative. At times she and her coworkers are supported by organizational resources from above (i.e., management, blunt end), and at other times they are challenged by the lack of what is needed for dealing with the situation at hand. Literature from other disciplines on decision-making in complex situations (e.g., airlines) supports the idea that RNs as workers in complex environments perform activities influenced by dynamic cognitive factors, including the knowledge they bring to the situation, their focus of attention or mindset, and the competing needs of patients, coworkers, and the organization. Nurses manage the context and complexity of actual care situations to prevent things from deteriorating as they anticipate, react, accommodate, adapt, and cope to reach decisions about care delivery in evolving situations. Recall Stella's description of knowing, hearing, and seeing and how she anticipated and prioritized. While the Cognitive Work of Nursing Framework (CWNF) is based on the Cognitive Work at the Sharp End of Practice framework and the "invisible work" it represents, it also includes concepts representing RN work at the sharp end such as clinical judgments and visible nursing care delivered.

What Do We Know About Nurse Knowing and Decision-making?

Using methods of direct observation and interviews with nurses, researchers have identified factors that contribute to the real life context and complexity of situations surrounding nursing practice (Ebright et al., 2003; Ebright et al., 2004; Benner et al., 2009; McGillis et al., 2010; Patterson et al., 2011; Sitterding et al., 2012; Sitterding et al., 2014). There is also abundant research regarding short- and long-term patient, nurse, and system outcomes of nursing care in relation to structural factors including patient and nurse characteristics and organizational characteristics (Aiken et al., 2014). Yet there continues to be a gap in knowledge and application of what we currently have evidence for related to the invisible or cognitive demands that influence RN clinical judgments. We have some evidence about how nurses in the context of actual care situations reach decisions about what and when care should be delivered through the invisible processes of clinical reasoning informed by cognitive stacking (Benner, 1999; Ebright et al., 2004; Potter et al., 2005; Sitterding et al., 2012,), and we have evidence about what nursing care is actually delivered (Kalisch et al., 2009). What is known is that the registered nurse on the front line is expected to perform within an attention-heavy dynamic and demanding work environment where the cognitive work is invisible and the stakes are extraordinarily high. What is necessary is a framework to understand factors influencing the cognitive work of nursing.

A Framework Describing the Cognitive Work of Nursing

Six major concepts are included in the Cognitive Work of Nursing Framework (CWNF): work complexity contributors; clinical reasoning-in-transition; cognitive stacking; clinical judgments; nursing care delivery; and patient, nurse, and system outcomes (see Table 1). In addition, three sub-concepts are included because of their important influence on clinical reasoning-in-transition in the context of actual RN work situations. These include situational awareness, knowledge in context, and managing competing goals.

The proposed framework represents the invisible cognitive work and the visible outcomes of that cognitive work for the individual RN in real-life care situations. As such, the framework is intended to reflect a dynamic systems approach to explanation of RN work and is aligned with complexity science principles (Lindberg et al., 2008). The foundation for complexity science is based on principles from several disciplines to explain how multiple systems evolve and maintain order. Complexity science principles can be used to understand and explain actual nursing care delivery to one patient within the larger context of an assignment, within a unit, within a department, or within a team. Complexity science can also be used to frame the multiple dynamic relationships that interact, adapt, and result in outcomes. In the CWNF, RN work is conceptualized as the RN representing a complex adaptive system (CAS) in relation to other CASs in the same or interacting care situations that result in the delivery of nursing care and

TABLE 1. **Cognitive Work of Nursing Framework Concepts and Definitions**

Framework concept	Definition
Work complexity contributors	Actual demands in the practice field that affect the behavioral and cognitive care delivery work of registered nurses, i.e., operational failures, design flaws, inadequate communication, complicated or irrelevant policies, and task management.
Clinical reasoning in transition	Practice reasoning over a specific period for multiple patients'/families' needs and problems, and informed by obvious and subtle changes in the dynamic surrounding environment; dependent upon management of competing goals, knowledge in context, and situational awareness.
Cognitive stacking	Cognitive workload management decision-making strategy for dealing with multiple care delivery requirements; mental list of to-be-done tasks; fail-sensitive strategy for preventing error or minimizing negative outcomes; discriminator between novice and expert nurses.
Clinical judgment	Interpretations or conclusions relevant to patient needs, concerns, or health problems and/or the decisions to: take action (or not), use or modify a standard approach, improvise new approach as deemed necessary by patient response/practice field demands.
Nursing care delivery	As a result of clinical judgment made in the context of actual practice situation and include activities and interventions implemented by a registered nurse and delegated to other providers by the registered nurse.
Situational awareness	Dynamic process of RN's *perception* with each cue relevant to patient concerns, issues, constraints and resources at any given time; *comprehension of their meaning* influencing a sense of salience; and the *anticipated projection* of their status in the near future influencing cognitive stacking and nursing care actions.
Knowledge in context	Knowledge that a direct care registered nurse brings to the situation. How the direct care nurse's knowledge informs him/her about what to expect with what they see and/or are experiencing.
Managing competing goals	Informs intent to act and decision-making and includes conflicts, resolution, and trade-offs. Cognitive task management: what needs to be done first and what can wait.

outcomes of that care. We know what clinical judgments should drive care delivery in a perfect and linear world. What we know less about is what transpires to influence clinical judgments about care in a complex world (i.e., the invisible cognitive work), nor how to support RNs effectively and reliably in this work. CWNF concepts and relationships are presented to guide understanding and support of RN work, both visible and invisible, through design of structural and system processes.

In the proposed CWNF, the RN interacts within a healthcare environment that includes complex processes and structures (e.g., layout of the care unit, location of medications, process for obtaining and receiving lab specimens and results, other individual care providers and teams). Work complexity contributors are environmental demands that arise within and across healthcare systems, such as the communications and task management activities described by Stella in the case study. The RN continuously interacts with multiple environmental demands while at the same time using constantly adapting clinical reasoning (clinical reasoning-in-transition) to evaluate patient situations and alternative care options.

The real-life care situation requires a constant state of attention to the unexpected. The RN needs the ability to clinically reason-in-transition continuously throughout care delivery, noticing and attending to multiple, sometimes subtle, cues about changing patient data and environmental conditions and demands. Information processing and vulnerability to the possibility of cognitive or information overload is real. The cognitive work of clinical reasoning illustrates RN information processing.

Three factors are essential for understanding clinical reasoning by RNs in actual care situations: situational awareness, knowledge (in context), and management of competing goals. Through a process called cognitive stacking, the RN continuously adapts to and copes with care delivery challenges related to prioritization and ordering of care needs, managing competing organizational and personal goals in the context of work complexity to arrive at clinical judgments regarding *what* nursing care to deliver and *how* it will be delivered (Ebright, 2003) (see Figure 1). The resulting nursing care that is delivered leads to outcomes that have implications for patients/families, nurses, and/or organizational system(s). Stella describes the various information inputs (alarms, patients, coworkers) and how she processes, manages, and stacks information.

> *There had been a pump going off in my patient's room. Before, as I was walking into the med room, I looked in there. He was in isolation so I could have either chosen to garb-up, go in and address it, ungarb, go out, go in the med room and get my meds. He was not bothered by the pump. I told him, "I'm getting your other medications, I'll be in in just a minute." And other nurses in the unit just left it beeping. While I was in the med room another nurse heard that beeping, went to see what was going on, and it was an amiodarone drip. It was this nurse that interrupted me. She just wanted to confirm with me that it was okay to add volume and to continue running it. That's all. I didn't log out of*

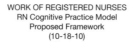

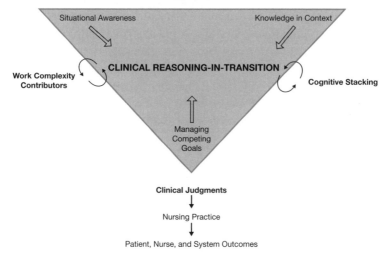

(copyright P. Ebright and M. Sitterding, 2010)

FIGURE 1. **Cognitive Work of Nursing Framework Overview**

the Pyxis or anything. I allowed the interruption, had the conversation and then resumed. I wanted to make sure that everything was okay ... that my patient was stable, that my patient was getting the medication the he was supposed to receive.

—Nurse, 2–5 years experience

Framework Concepts

These concepts are: work complexity contributors; clinical reasoning-in-transition; knowledge in context; situational awareness; management of competing goals; cognitive stacking; clinical judgments; nursing practice; and patient, nurse, and system outcomes.

Work Complexity Contributors

"Work complexity contributors" are a major concept in the model and are defined as the actual demands in the practice field that affect the behavioral and cognitive work of RNs.

Studies on the actual practice of nursing have reported numerous complexity work contributors that challenge the successful management of work that is essential for safe and quality care (Bittner, 2009; Ebright, 2003; Krichbaum et al., 2007; Potter et al., 2005; Hall et al., 2010; Lindberg, 2008). The most frequently reported work complexity contributors influencing nursing practice include equipment/supply issues, flawed facility or structural design, inadequate communication/documentation processes, inadequate staffing or staffing mix patterns, complex medication management processes, complicated or irrelevant policies, and response time to requests for information or support (Cornell et al., 2010). For example, in one study (Tucker, 2004) the remarkable impact of system failures on nursing work was observed among 26 nurses within nine hospitals where 194 system failures were observed (on average one failure every 74 minutes at an estimated cost of $117.00/failure). The average nurse was found to complete 84 nursing tasks per shift, with tasks taking an average of 3.1 minutes per task and the nurse switching, or cognitively shifting, between patients every 11 minutes and being interrupted mid-task up to eight times per shift (Tucker, 2008). In another study of 27 nurses over a four-week period during actual work and 98.2 hours of observation that 77% of each of the recorded activities by nurses lasted less than 30 seconds, demonstrating the frequent shifting of nurse activities (Cornell et al., 2010). The investigators described the nature of the work activities as "back-and-forth," and rarely completed without interruption and switching cognitive focus or thinking from one aspect of care to another.

Management of cognitive shifts is inherent in the current practice of nursing care delivery (Sitterding et al., 2014). The work complexity contributors described above represent some of the *problem parameters* of the care delivery situations in which nurses find themselves on a daily basis. Problem parameters are those characteristics or attributes of a problematic situation that require interpretation for problem-solving. Problem parameters are important to understand for the challenges they present to clinical reasoning and to subsequent judgments about appropriate care and how to deliver it in clinical situations encountered by RNs. Patterson and colleagues (2010) reported finding the six following examples of problem parameters, or attributes of clinical situations, reported by RNs:

1. Competing goals
2. Unpredictability
3. Clinical urgency

4. Time constraints
5. Duration demanded by an activity
6. Lack of control

The following represents Stella's consideration of problem parameters in making a decision about when to respond to certain cues.

> *I mean, it really depends I guess, it depends on what it is, you know, that I have to finish. If it's baths, in terms of me walking back from, you know I administer a med and I gotta get back to the computer to make sure I document the med has been given cause you know what'll happen if I don't get back to the computer and document that the med's been given: the icon will pop up. Some nurse trying to help me out will see that the med's not been given and then they'll go give the med again. Patient will get a double dose. I get interrupted going back from the patient's room to the desk and if I get interrupted, if it's fast, you know, um, I might just take care of it. I might help 'em out and then just really quickly get back to, you know, charting. However, putting patients on the bedside commode, that's not fast. Patients wanting a pain med, that's not fast. Something for comfort, you know, can I get a blanket, yes, that's fast, I can quickly do that. And, you know, and get back to the computer. Getting a cup of water, that's fast. Getting a blanket, that's fast. If it's fast, I'll take care of it. But helping the ambulance crew, that's not fast. But if it's urgent I will stop. I will absolutely stop what I'm doin' and help the ambulance crew cause they gotta get back on, they gotta get back on the street.*
>
> —Expert Nurse

Clinical Reasoning-in-Transition

The second major concept in the proposed framework, clinical reasoning-in-transition, is dependent on the processes of critical thinking and problem-solving imposed by ongoing and dynamic work complexity contributors encountered by the RN throughout actual care delivery.

Clinical reasoning has been defined as " ... the processes by which nurses and other clinicians make their judgments, and includes both the deliberate process of generating alternatives, weighing them against the evidence, and choosing the most appropriate, and those patterns that might be characterized as engaged, practical reasoning" (Tanner et al., 2006).

Reasoning-in-transition has been defined as "practical reasoning where a clinician takes account of gains and losses in understanding a situation as transitions occur" (Benner et al., 1999). Other definitions of clinical reasoning are similar in their focus on problem-solving for patient needs by clinicians (Fonteyn 2000; Hawkins et al., in press).

The use of the term "clinical reasoning-in-transition" in the CWNF was chosen to emphasize an additional purpose and focus for most, if not all, decision-making that RNs do while in the midst of actual care delivery situations, or the meeting of expectations inherent in managing work flow bounded by a specific time period or shift.

We propose that even judgments about order and priority of work activities are imbedded in the reasoning about clinical indicators of patient status and needs at any point in time. Judgments about organizing and prioritizing are influenced by generating alternatives about timing and degree of completeness of delivering care activities across multiple patients and environmental demands, and by the effect of those judgments on safety and quality. Clinical reasoning-in-transition requires the ability to notice subtle changes in a patient's condition over time as well as in the context of environmental demands. We have found that clinical reasoning-in-transition in actual work situations is clinical reasoning over a specific time period for multiple patients' and families' needs and problems, and is informed by obvious and subtle changes in the dynamic surrounding environment, including status of coworkers and team members (Patterson et al., 2013). As such, clinical reasoning-in-transition is pertinent to the safe and effective delivery of care to individual and groups of patients, and includes management of workflow.

In the CWNF, the effectiveness of clinical reasoning-in-transition is informed by three important cognitive factors that determine how practitioners deliver care: knowledge in context, situational awareness, and management of competing goals.

Knowledge in Context
Knowledge in context relates to the process by which practitioners use knowledge effectively in actual work situations (Cook et al., 1994). Three aspects of knowledge in context are important to consider for understanding the challenges relative to RNs using knowledge when and where

needed. These aspects include the knowledge that RNs bring to the situation, how the RNs organize their knowledge to make inferences about what is happening and what they expect to happen, and the extent to which knowledge can be activated in a specific situation.

Knowledge on-hand for managing clinical situations depends on, in addition to the RN's individual cognitive capacity, their education and previous experiences, as well as information available in the actual situation. Types of knowledge reported by RNs to influence their decision-making while delivering care include knowledge about specific patient disease conditions (e.g., symptoms of myocardial infarctions), knowledge unique to individual patients (e.g., that the patient is blind and needs assistance with medications), as well as knowledge about unit routines and staff (e.g., that physician rounds are usually completed by 10AM, or Robert RN is great to work with).

How well the RN organizes information effectively for situations encountered depends on the completeness and accuracy of information and/or on the knowledge available and accessible. Practitioners organize information into mental models or representations to make inferences about the current situation (Klein, 1998). In a situation in which the RN has inadequate knowledge due to inexperience or to inaccurate or missing information, misunderstanding of the situation may occur, resulting in subsequent decisions that lead to unintended outcomes. For example, a nurse's judgment to resuscitate an elderly terminal patient as a result of inaccessible information on code status may result in poor outcomes for the patient, the patient's family, and the healthcare team. The RN may have had no alternative in the actual work situation, however, given the information available and the urgency of the situation.

The third aspect of knowledge in context is the ability "to call it to mind when it is relevant to the problem at hand and whether he or she knows how to use this knowledge in problem-solving" (Cook et al., 1994). Although having an accurate mental model or representation of a situation is crucial for effective intervention, maintaining and correcting representations are also essential for the dynamic situations encountered by RNs in delivery of clinical care. Cognitive work is evident in the nurse who is constantly problem-solving by adding, subtracting, and reordering priorities as patients or work conditions and system failures (work complexity contributors) warrant. Partitioning (bundling tasks among several patients), interweaving (providing care for multiple patients in cyclical fashion), and reprioritization (continually adapting work plans) were identified as care management strategies used by nurses to manage their workload (Tucker, 2006).

Situational Awareness

Situational awareness, the second cognitive factor affecting clinical reasoning-in-transition and a sub-concept in the model, is imperative for accurate decision-making in the midst of frequent cognitive shifts. The contribution of the knowledge-in-context factors (content, organization, and activation) is dependent on the RN's situational awareness in a given care delivery situation. It was suggested that situational awareness is the most influential factor influencing control of attention (Cook et al., 1994). Situational awareness is an internalized mental model of the current state in a dynamic environment (Klein, 1998). It is "being aware of all that is occurring in the situation and what might be causing it" (Bogner, 1994). More specifically, behavioral and cognitive stages influencing situational awareness include: (1) noticing events in a dynamic environment; (2) assigning meaning to what is noticed; and (3) predicting or projecting the implications of what is noticed (Bogner, 1994). In nursing, situational awareness is defined as "a dynamic process in which a nurse perceives each clinical cue relevant to the patient and his or her environment; comprehends and assigns meaning to those cues resulting in a patient-centric sense of salience; and projects or anticipates required interventions based on those cues" (Sitterding et al., 2012). It is the product of individual capabilities, experiences, goal-driven behaviors, informational environments, and resource constraints (Endsley, 2000).

Inability to control attention can result in failure to notice something about the current situation (inattentional blindness), or the failure to notice that something is different (change blindness). Both types of failures in attention can affect RNs noticing or responding to changes in patient conditions and/or their anticipation of subsequent trajectories and how to manage them. When quick action is the central focus in a clinical situation (i.e., situations of criticality in nursing, such as the pediatric nurse in the midst of environmental challenges and faced with a critically ill child), interpretation of the situation rather than choices for action is the core phenomenon with implications for patient safety and quality. Interpretation is about making sense of blurred images, in essence multiple pieces of sensory information at one time culminating into an issue the nurse needs to address—or not. Researchers highlight the significance of surveillance and its concomitant interpretation of the significance of weak as well as strong signals as a key competency for nurses (Benner et al., 1999). Expert situational awareness is illustrated as Stella describes her surveillance habits.

> *You always look in your rooms, whether they're your patients or not because you never know what you're gonna see. Walking by you can see a number of things. For example, you might be walking by a patient's room, not your patient, but you still check it out. We're all here for the same thing and that's patient care ... and one of our main concerns is their safety. So, for example, I might be walking by a patient's room that's not mine, and they might be leaning over their bed as far as they can trying to reach something on the floor. I'm thinking "Oh, hey, what are you trying to get? Let me help with that," and you go in there and you get it and you hand it to them. And that keeps your, whoever's patient, just that patient in general, it keeps them from possibly losing their balance, falling out of bed on their head—safety. Or you might walk by and see that a patient's desatting, and it could be something as simple as they're simply fidgeting or they're scratching their head, or they've taken their O_2 monitor off. It could be just a number of things. So I always look when I go by because you just never know when they may need your help.*
>
> —Expert Nurse

The proposed framework depicts a relationship between situational awareness and clinical reasoning-in-transition. Further, relationships between work complexity contributors and situational awareness are also described since environmental demands such as interruptions discussed earlier may distract the RN from accurate interpretation of a situation and result in faulty decision-making as a result of information overload.

Management of Competing Goals

Management of competing goals informs intentions to act and make decisions, and includes conflicts, resolutions, and trade-offs. Trade-offs represent how the RN copes with different goals that conflict in the midst of uncertainty, risk, and the pressure of limited resources (Cook et al., 1994). Managing competing goals captures the clinical reasoning-in-transition and resulting judgments around what needs to be done first for safety, quality, and efficient workflow, what can wait, and to what extent care delivery activities can be performed according to organizational and/or personal standards given the complexity of the situation. For example, the RN who wants to provide pain medication for a patient, respond to a team member who has requested help with a patient transfer, and needs to take a phone call from a physician regarding discharge orders for another patient, must make judgments about which goal to accomplish first in the context of the uncertainty, risk, and limited resources surrounding these competing goals. This illustrates the concept of information overload and management. The judgment may involve trade-offs about what may have to be postponed to move forward on what the RN decides is the most important goal.

Personal goals also may compete with patient care and organizational goals. This is particularly salient for new graduate nurses. A new graduate may be conflicted about whether to perform according to standards learned in school or to adopt the routines the RN perceives as universally accepted by his or her new colleagues on the care unit he or she has joined. Research suggests a relationship between the self-generated and sometimes externally generated social pressure experienced by new graduates and its impact on their care delivery judgments (Ebright et al., 2004). A study of RNs' competing goals that were operating in specific care delivery situations revealed goal patterns that fell into five categories (Ebright et al., 2003):

1. Maintain patient safety
2. Get everything done to prevent getting behind
3. Avoid increasing complexity
4. Appear competent and efficient to coworkers
5. Maintain patient/family satisfaction and patient flow

Maintaining patient safety and patient/family satisfaction as part of the goals of RNs seem very clear and consistent with what healthcare customers and administrators desire. Three of the other goals are related to organization and completion of work (prevent getting behind, avoid increasing complexity, maintain patient flow) and reflect challenging aspects of the clinical reasoning-in-transition process that is bound by a specific time period. Attainment of all the other goals will, to some extent, determine accomplishment of the remaining goal: appearing competent and efficient to coworkers. Traditional nursing education and continuing education have focused on those goals related to clinical care. Students learn about organizing and finishing work in the context of competing goals primarily after completing their basic programs and during orientation and the first year of practice. Consider the bi-directional relationship between information overload and the nurse's ability to manage competing goals as Stella's coworker describes the challenge to manage information and completing goals.

> *My phone rings every five minutes regardless of what I'm doing ... I might be trying to check a chart. I'm helping a patient. I'm giving medicine. I'm talking with a student nurse, if I'm fortunate enough to have one that I'm working with that day ... It could be the unit secretary saying, "Patient 42 wants ice." Or, they need to go to the bathroom or they need pain meds. Or it could be the PIC team, and it happened to me this morning, calling me saying, "Is there any reason this patient can't have a line in his arm?" I wasn't even in that patient's room! How can I see what's going on? It's very difficult, to be honest. I very nearly always answer the phone. The only times that I don't are when the battery goes dead. The battery tends to go dead about 11 AM. It's just really hard to always know what's going on.*
>
> —Nurse (<2 years' experience)

The clear decision about what intervention is best for the patient, or how best to provide an intervention, competes with workflow goals. And if these goal patterns challenge clinical reasoning-in-transition in experienced RNs, how much more strongly do they influence the ability of student nurses and new graduates to manage care delivery safely and accurately? The student and new graduate do not readily observe and see clearly how experienced RNs accomplish the cognitive work needed to resolve conflicting and competing goals. In fact, most experienced RNs manage these situations invisibly and effortlessly (Ebright et al., 2003).

Cognitive Stacking

The third major concept in the proposed model is *cognitive stacking*. How the nurse decides to cognitively stack is directly related to the nurse's ability to interpret the salience of information content and information flow. Like work complexity contributors, there is a dynamic and reciprocal relationship between cognitive stacking and clinical reasoning-in-transition. Cognitive stacking was defined as a process in terms of the following four characteristics (Ebright et al., 2003):

1. A cognitive workload management decision-making strategy for dealing with multiple care delivery requirements
2. A mental list of multiple to-do tasks
3. A failure-sensitive strategy for preventing error and/or minimizing bad outcomes
4. A discriminator between novice and experienced RN practice

In addition to RN experience, the effectiveness (breadth, depth, and efficiency) of cognitive stacking and their resulting decisions we propose are dependent on the ability of the RN to maintain situational awareness or on the extent to which the RN could be mindful and make sense of clinical and workflow data throughout dynamic situations (Ebright et al., 2003). As such, cognitive stacking is closely and continuously aligned to clinical reasoning-in-transition, both for its dependence on and its informing of clinical reasoning-in-transition work. Information processing through cognitive stacking results in eight different types of decisions: defer, shed, reorder, complete, recruit, cluster, be proactive, and reduce performance criteria.

These workflow management decisions were often found to be important for preventing complications or patient deterioration, and for minimizing apparent problems already in progress. For example, an RN describes deciding to defer care activities that would require continuous attention and availability until team resources are accessible to cover other patients in her assignment. An RN reports making the decision to interrupt current flow of care to complete a task or procedure that is important and, if delayed, might be difficult to fit into the work flow and complexity they anticipate for later in the shift. In other words, as a result of anticipation of workflow changes and their potential impact and consequence for clinical aspects of patient care, the RN decides to be proactive to avoid and minimize hazards or chaos later on.

Clinical Judgments

The fourth major concept in the CWNF is clinical judgments. Clinical judgment is defined by Tanner (2006) as "an interpretation or conclusion about a patient's needs, concerns, or health problems, and/or the decision to take action (or not), use or modify standard approaches, or improvise new ones as deemed appropriate by the patient's response." Tanner's definition is consistent with other literature (Facione, 2008), which proposed that clinical judgments were decisions about what to believe and/or do about a clinical situation. For the purpose of the CWNF and to more clearly reflect the nature of actual practice bound by time and setting, we propose minor modification to Tanner's definition as follows: the concept of clinical judgments is defined as interpretation or conclusion about patient needs, concerns, or health problems, and/or the decision to take action (or not), use or modify standard approaches, or improvise new ones as deemed appropriate by patient responses and practice field demands.

Clinical judgments result from clinical reasoning-in-transition; thus, in this model, they are the products of critical thinking and problem-solving involving patient needs and concerns, as well as critical thinking and problem-solving surrounding dynamic work complexity contributors and cognitive stacking. Clinical judgments for the purpose of the proposed framework incorporate the recommendation to shift from a focus on critical thinking to multiple ways of thinking, by supporting the belief that critical thinking is necessary, but alone is insufficient for nursing practice (Kalish et al., 2009).

In addition, clinical judgments result from clinical reasoning-in-transition complicated by challenges to maintaining situational awareness, application of knowledge in context, and managing competing goals.

Nursing Practice
The fifth major concept in the proposed model is nursing practice. Nursing practice is defined as those activities and interventions implemented by an RN, or delegated to other providers by an RN, as a result of clinical judgments made in the context of actual practice situations. Nursing practice includes all activities actually performed or delegated by an RN resulting from clinical judgments about what care is needed, when care is needed, and how to best deliver the care given the demands of the practice field. Examples of nursing practice would include direct care activities such as vital sign monitoring, dressing changes, assessments, mobilization, pain management, and medication administration. Other nursing practice examples include stress management and education provided on chronic disease management, and the care provided by others through delegation and direction from the RN.

In addition to those activities and interventions implemented, the CWNF also takes into account the activities and interventions identified as needed in a care situation by standards and guidelines for practice, but not delivered in the actual situation. For example, protocols for pressure ulcer management in an organization may call for routine position adjust-ment, but the care is not delivered because the patient is unavailable (a work complexity contributor), workflow overload precludes staff attention to the care needed (requiring cognitive stacking), or there is a care provider performance problem (knowledge in context, work complexity contrib-utor). While deficiencies in nursing practice may be due to lack of skills and easily remediated, understanding judgments leading to the care not being delivered is essential for making lasting improvements.

Patient, Nurse, and System Outcomes
The sixth major concept in the CWNF is patient, nurse, and system outcomes. Outcomes within the model represent: the patient (nurse-sen-sitive outcomes), the nurse (nursing satisfaction and engagement), and the environment (benchmarking system performance in people, safety, quality, innovation, and finance). Although patient outcomes are linked to organizational structures in acute care, there is growing evidence that process variables related to nursing surveillance, quality of the working environment, and quality of interaction with other professionals lead to differences among hospitals on mortality and complication rates (refer-ence). These process variables often reflect the actual work of nursing regardless of nursing role or type of organizational setting. Using a human factors framework (e.g., Operating at the Sharp End of Practice Framework), these process variables and their relationships to clinical judgments, nursing practice, and resulting patient, nurse, and system outcomes can be examined to understand the complex and multifaceted aspects of the actual practice of RNs.

This examination of processes should include the complex cognitive work of RNs and the effect of the demands of the environment on RN cognitive work and resulting outcomes, in addition to the organizational structures that best support that work and relate to information overload in nurses. Research outcomes in health care have grown tremendously over the last two decades as expectations of healthcare system accountability have increased (Doran, 2010). Research related to mortality and other adverse outcomes has shown these outcomes to be linked to organizational struc-tures such as staffing and staff mix, rather than process variables (Aiken et al., Needleman et al.). We propose that outcomes dependent on nursing practice are the result of the visible and invisible cognitive work of nursing. Understanding the concepts and concept relationships represented in the

CWNF will likely result in enhanced design of care delivery systems and environments and nursing education to support this RN work.

Tips and Tools for Applying the RN Practice Framework

The CWNF is a useful guide when considering factors influencing patient safety and quality. Acknowledging the critical contribution of knowledge in context to clinical reasoning-in-transition would be manifested, for example, by thinking creatively about best care delivery models and processes that account for appropriate assignment and continuous support of all RNs who have to care for unfamiliar patient populations. Another example is creative thinking about best care delivery models and processes that provide appropriate assignment and continuous support for new graduates and less experienced RNs with less knowledge about critical, yet subtle, clinical cues signaling patient deterioration, or complex situations requiring reorganization of priorities. In support of the new graduate or the experienced RN transitioning to a new unit or practice area, consider the following: (1) Simulations requiring the development and cognitive use of surveillance habits; and (2) Pairing expert nurses with non-expert nurses to enable situational coaching, allowing the non-expert nurse to observe the expert nurse using clinical reasoning-in-transition; staffing and scheduling that take into account that non-expert nurses will be more prone to inattention and change blindness.

Another approach to maximize the cognitive work of the RN is to enable the voice of the RN in innovative environmental designs that decrease distractions about care delivery such as: reliable resource availability that eliminates hunting for and waiting on needed supplies or equipment; reliable, easy, and immediate access to medications, intravenous fluids, and supplies. Other environmental designs to enhance situational awareness would be those that increase the availability of information and cues to inform clinical reasoning-in-transition. For example, unit structural designs that maximize the visibility both of locations and the statuses of other team members so that RNs can assess the human resources available to assist them, or evaluate the needs of other team members (for example, new graduates and less experienced RNs). Consider situational awareness pitfalls described in Chapter 1 and how to combat them:

1. **Attention tunneling**—Creating good situational awareness depends on one's ability to switch attention between different sources of information. Consider simulation scenarios that enable attention switching.

2. **Memory trap**—Avoid an over-reliance on memory.

3. **Workload and fatigue**—Acknowledge and act upon the impact of workload and fatigue on situational awareness. Identify and eliminate factors (worked hours, effective delegation, team members' recognition of one another's fatigue levels) contributing to workload and fatigue.

4. **Data overload**—Consider the relationship between cognitive workflow and the use of the electronic health records (EHR). Identify and eliminate unnecessary technology data points within one's hospital setting.

Those involved in the design of structures and processes in which RNs deliver care would demonstrate acknowledgment of the challenge of managing competing goals and its impact on clinical reasoning-in-transition by eliminating those expectations of RNs that do not contribute directly to the safe, quality care of patients. Introduction of new initiatives or processes that interrupt care delivery, or add additional steps to a process that is not intended to improve direct care, should be evaluated before implementation for the extent to which they have the potential to compete with important direct care goals. The focus on consumer satisfaction scores, outcome indicators, and the link to value-based purchasing has resulted in much redesign and process improvement activities. Attention to the effect of these new initiatives, and their design and implementation, on both the visible and invisible work of RNs is essential for maintaining and making improvements in quality and patient safety. Consider an interview process (Klein, 2003; Sitterding et al., 2014) enabling one to discover the cognitive work of competing goals.

The process of cognitive stacking is demonstrated by avoidance of retrospective narrow and linear assessment of error events, and/or criticism of judgments made by nurses about the care of individual patient situations. RN complex work in the context of actual care situations is laden with demands for clinical judgments surrounding and dependent on patient(s), team member(s), unit environment, and time boundaries. The cognitive stacking work required to inform the clinical reasoning-in-transition resulting in best judgments is not simple or linear.

Acknowledging clinical judgments as proposed in this framework as an outcome of clinical reasoning-in-context assumes that judgments result from a process involving multiple factors, and are often dependent on contextual factors nxot obviously related to a simple right or wrong decision. For example, believing that lack of a certain piece of knowledge (such as the policy related to the specific situation and judgment) was the reason for a poor outcome—and that therefore education is the appropriate solution for improvement—discounts all of the RN cognitive work surrounding the situation and influencing clinical reasoning-in-transition that resulted in the judgment. The data often not collected and overlooked but needed to make improvements in outcomes is that related to the clinical reasoning-in-transition resulting in the judgment. Policies rarely address context.

Understanding and Applying the CWNF: Consider the Situation in Context

Understanding and applying the CWNF requires one to understand the situation-in-context. Contextual factors might include staffing mix, unit culture, relationship between the care delivery team members, competing and complex demands within the nursing work environment, the patient's condition, nursing assignments, and nursing expertise. Three principles to consider include the following:

1. Continuously changing contextual factors challenges the ability of the RN to attend to the present situation.
2. Contextual factors inform judgments and decisions about the prioritization of care for patient safety and quality outcomes.
3. These contextual factors contain critical information for care that leads to multiple and competing RN goals.

References

Aiken, L. H., Smith, H. L., & Lake, E. T. (1994). Lower Medicare mortality among a set of hospitals known for good nursing care. *Medical Care, 32*(8), 771–787.

Benner, P., Tanner, C. A., & Chesla, C. A. (2009). *Expertise in nursing practice: Caring, clinical judgment, and ethics* (2nd ed.). New York, NY: Springer Publishing.

Benner, P. (1999). *From novice to expert: Excellence and power in clinical nursing practice.* Menlo Park, CA: Addison-Wesley.

Cook, R. I., & Woods, D. D. (1994). Operating at the sharp end: The complexity of human error. In Edward Boger (Ed.), *Human Error in Medicine* (225–310). Hillsdale, NJ: Lawrence Erlbaum Associates.

Ebright, P., Urden, L., Patterson, E., & Chalko, B. (2004). Themes surrounding novice nurse near-miss and adverse event situations. *Journal of Nursing Administration, 34,* 11.

Endsley, M. R., & Garland, D. J. (2000). *Situational awareness analysis and measurement.* Mahwah, NJ: Lawrence Erlbaum Associates.

Endsley, M. R., & Garland, D. J. (2000). Theoretical underpinnings of situational awareness: A critical review. In M. R. Endsley & D. J. Garland (Eds.), *Situational awareness analysis and measurement* (3–32). Mahwah, NJ: Lawrence Erlbaum Associates.

Facione, Noreen C. & Facione, Peter A. (2008). Critical thinking and clinical judgment. In Noreen C. Facione & Peter A. Facione (Eds.), *Critical Thinking and Clinical Reasoning in the Health Sciences: A Teaching Anthology* (1–13). Millbrae, CA: California Academic Press.

Fonteyn, M. E., & Fisher, A. (1995). Use of think aloud method to study nurses' reasoning and decision making in clinical practice settings. *Journal of Neuroscience Nursing, 27,* 124–128.

Hall, L. M., Pedersen, C., Hubley, P., Ptack, E., Hemingway, A., Watson, C., & Keatings, M. (2010). Interruptions and pediatric patient safety. *Journal of Pediatric Nursing* 25, 167–75.

Kalisch, B., Landstrom, G., & Williams, R. (2009). Missed nursing care: Errors of omission. *Nursing Outlook, 57*(1), 3–9.

Klein, G. (1998). *Sources of power: How people make decisions.* Cambridge, MA: MIT Press.

Krichbaum, K., Diemert, C., Jacox, L., Jones, A., Koenig, P., Mueller, C. & Disch, J. (2007). Complexity compression: Nurses under fire. *Nursing Forum, 42*(2), 86–94.

McGillis-Hall, L., Pedersen, C., Hubley, P., Ptack, E., Hemingway, A., Watson, C., & Keatings, M. (2008). Interruptions and pediatric patient safety. *Journal of Pediatric Nursing, 25,* 167–175.

McGillis Hall, L., Pedersen, C., & Fairley, L. (2010). Losing the moment: Understanding interruptions to nurses' work. *Journal of Nursing Association, 40*(4), 169–176.

Needleman, J., Buerhaus, P., Mattke, S., Steward, M., & Zelevinsky, K. (2002). Nurse-staffing levels and the quality of care in hospitals. *New England Journal of Medicine, 346*(22), 1715–1722.

Potter, P., Boxerman, S., Dunagan, C., et al. (2005). Understanding the cognitive work of nursing in the acute care environment. *Journal of Nursing Administration, 3,* 327–335.

Patterson, E. S., Ebright, P., & Saleem, J. (2011). Investigating stacking: How do registered nurses prioritize their activities in real time? *International Journal of Industrial Ergonomics, 41,* 389–393.

Sitterding, M., & Ebright, P. (2010). Patient safety and the cognitive work of nursing: Advanced in nursing science and implementations for organizational support. 43rd Annual Meeting. American Organization of Nurse Executives. Indianapolis, Indiana

3

Information Architecture

Timothy Tarnowski, MBA

"We shape our buildings; thereafter they shape us[.]"

—Winston Churchill

The quote above has been broadly interpreted to indicate that each of us take on characteristics of our facilities and buildings. It propose that architecture has a profound effect on those it touches. In this chapter, we will expand upon this theme of physical space by including technology used to take care of patients. The "architecture" of the various components in the patient care setting can also have a profound effect on the ability of those it touches to attend to important cues and information in their environment.

Today's healthcare delivery system has been built upon a highly complex "architecture" of interrelated components. These components include multi-disciplinary teams, physical space, clinical protocols, operating procedures, and technology. While these components are highly interrelated, they are often "architected" and implemented separately from one another.

These physical separations often lead to a sense of disconnectedness for patients and families. Patients, providers, and others involved in patient care have described processes that are fragmented, inefficient, ineffective, or unreliable. When processes work, the end results are achieved, but many times "workarounds" by staff are required to achieve the desired outcomes. Navigating the multitude of interrelated work processes with no clear roadmap can be a daunting challenge which results in frustrations on a daily basis for providers. These frustrations can adversely impact interactions with patients and their families.

As a result, most healthcare organizations have been working very hard to streamline processes for patients and their families. There are a number of organizational improvement process frameworks used in business, such as Lean Six Sigma, which attempts to reduce complexity and improve existing processes, reliability, efficiencies, and effectiveness. Some have even deployed these methods when designing new processes.

There are multiple factors at play in the healthcare setting which the providers and our patients need to navigate on a daily basis. These factors include physical space layout, the variety of team members who contribute to patient care, equipment, technology, and computer software. Each of these factors add to the complexity and burden in the healthcare setting. Generally, these components have been put together in a piecemeal approach, which can contribute to patient inconveniences and increase the burden on providers.

Karl E. Weick and Kathleen M. Sutcliffe, authors of the book *Managing the Unexpected* (2001), base their framework on a high-reliability organization (HRO) model. Many in the healthcare industry are pursuing this HRO model due to the complexity of the patient-care environment.

This chapter will examine the impact of multiple factors on patients, their families, and those involved in care-giving processes. The themes explored here can be applied to the full continuum of care.

Information Overload: Learning from Patients We Serve

Patients expect that they will be prepared for what will happen to them during hospitalizations, will have their questions answered, and that they will receive safe, high-quality care. When thinking about the impact of space, multiple healthcare team members, equipment, and computer software, we should start with the patients we serve. In this chapter, we begin with the patient at the center of a simple diagram. The circle in Figure 2 represents workflows and space.

We will then show how each component in the healthcare environment (space, multi-disciplinary team members, equipment, technology, and computer software) add to the complexity of the patient's experience and is a potential increase in the burden of the healthcare providers.

We will use this simple model to demonstrate the potential complexity of all the components interacting within the circle (space and workflow). Although we are including only some of the variables, the model will become visually complex. This visual complexity is intended to represent what patients, their families, and the multi-disciplinary team members face each day they interact.

Each of us has been a patient and experienced the various processes of contacting a healthcare provider organization, scheduling an appointment, going to the care location, being examined and treated, and then sent back to our homes. Patients approach healthcare organizations with various illnesses and concerns. They are often weary, and at times afraid of what the outcome of their visit might be.

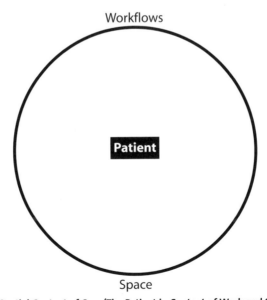

FIGURE 2. The Spatial Context of Care (The Patient in Context of Work and Space)

As patients approach a healthcare organization, they seek answers to medical questions or are looking for wellness advice. They often do not know where to start or what to ask. Our patient intake processes should be designed to be simple, clear, and efficient. Many patients start with a phone call. Our ability to quickly assess the situation and clearly advise the patient on their next move is a critical first step in the process. There are many necessary forms and requirements.

As patients interact with healthcare organizations, they encounter a variety of roles, and the information exchange becomes increasingly complex. With each person that enters into the equation, the complexity increases exponentially.

The diagram in Figure 3 maintains the patient at the center of the model. Each role within the healthcare organization increases the need for information exchange and process coordination. The arrows in the model indicate the increased number of information exchange points that are introduced with each role. The interactions do not occur exactly as diagramed, but this illustrates the increased potential for interactions as each role gets introduced into the model. This version is purposefully over-simplified, but illustrates the point that there are increasing complexities in interactions,

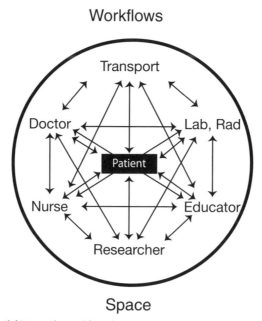

FIGURE 3. **Potential Interactions with Patient**

types of information required, and processing that patients experience as they attempt to negotiate the system.

Each of the roles included in the diagram has the potential to exchange data and information with every other role. As the levels of communication increase, the model becomes more complex. This is visually represented in that each role is connected with every other one. While it is not entirely accurate that each role will interact with every other role, there are multiple roles within each shape. The diagram in Figure 3 suggests how, over the course of their interaction with healthcare organizations, a patient might begin to feel a bit overwhelmed in the process. It is easy to see how the complexity of our interactions can impact the experience of our patients and their families. In addition, given the complexities of the number and type of interactions, it is also possible for errors in communication to occur between and among the individuals in this diagram.

Starting from the patient's perspective, as we work to provide clarity, we need to build our information gathering and sharing processes so that patients can easily understand and follow the necessary steps for their recovery. Today's patients are exposed to the Internet through smartphones, tablets, and a myriad of other technologies. They can, and often do, easily search for answers to their questions about retail, banking, travel, and any other services they are seeking. Comparison shopping is easy, convenient, and expected. These comparisons and expectations from patients and families are also becoming more commonplace in health care.

Patients expect that they will be prepared for what will happen to them during hospitalizations (i.e., procedures), will have their questions answered, and that they will receive safe, high-quality care. Healthcare organizations have made some significant strides in this direction, yet have much work to do. Patients have come to expect rapid, clear, and easy access to data and information. Health care is not exempt from these expectations, and as we create our physical space and workflows we need to be mindful of these expectations.

Space Design Considerations

Undoubtedly, physical space impacts our approaches and behaviors on a daily basis. Physical space and workflow are represented in the model as the circle surrounding the patient and the various roles of providers in the healthcare system. Space and workflow introduce new elements that need to be factored into the interactions in order to increase the efficiency and effectiveness of our healthcare environment. Older facilities introduce both patients and providers to different experiences than newer spaces. Virtual interactions (defined as electronic communications) using smartphone or video conferencing between any members of the care team have impacted the physical space requirements and considerations for healthcare organizations. For instance, providers can communicate face-to-face using electronic communication devices without physically being in the same location. These types of electronic interactions may impact space design where providers traditionally gathered to do their work.

Many healthcare facilities were designed decades ago, before the current protocols, operating procedures, and technology were even under consideration. Older healthcare facilities place patients in smaller rooms which may impede the providers' ability to interact with the patients and their families due to current space needs for technology and monitoring equipment, among other things.

At several different organizations, newly constructed facilities have replaced aging inpatient facilities. Clinical units have been relocated from aging inpatient facilities, which were limited in size and capabilities. The staff had to interact in very close quarters and certainly became highly skilled in adapting to their space limitations. They also got to know each other very well due to the close working conditions. The aging buildings certainly shaped their relationships with each other, their interactions with their patients and families, as well as their ability to assess their patients' conditions and needs.

Overall, the aging space was considered acceptable. However, providers often commented that the space seemed to be the minimum necessary to properly care for patients. In these spaces, the providers had a small central work station where they would congregate to start their shift, transition from the previous shift's team, and then head out to the various patient rooms outside of the central work stations.

The professional providers frequently reported that conditions were pretty congested in the hallways and/or in the patient rooms. This impacted the interactions and movement of team members, patients, and equipment. Often times, there was not even enough space to accommodate some of the core services, such as: lab, radiology, therapies, environmental services, and even dieticians and pharmacy techs who work very hard to support the patients and providers. As a result, providers had to become extremely resourceful in their team interactions and their abilities to take care of their patients. The space became especially congested when visiting family members were seeking to spend time with their loved ones in the hospital.

While the healthcare providers found themselves in a familiar but aging facility, their environment was constantly evolving due to changes in regulations, clinical protocols, and advancing technology. Although the aging facility was shaping the behavior of providers and their interactions with each other as well as with their patients, providers found themselves in a continuously changing environment with increasing pressures. These pressures included, among numerous others, the need for increased documentation, alerts from most new clinical devices, and the multitude of new processes introduced by electronic medical records.

There were some advantages the providers expressed about their environment. As mentioned above, they were familiar with it. They each had developed ways to get their work done and provide the best care for their patients. For example, in very close quarters, the providers could easily communicate with each other since they were usually within sight or speaking distance of one another.

When a multi-disciplinary team has worked together in close quarters, they develop an operating rhythm and become very effective at collaborating together. This proximity can provide significant advantages for high-performing teams. However, this type of an environment can work against newly-forming teams, teams that are experiencing significant turnover, or teams with inexperienced team members who may struggle in less-than-optimal work space.

In several instances, the teams design their new facilities, including redesigning their workflows and adding the latest clinical and information technologies. For example, the new monitors, clinical devices, and even smart beds have the potential to provide relevant clinical data to the providers. Adding this modern equipment requires workflow redesign to leverage the benefits of the alerting capabilities. If this is not considered, then contemporary workflows leveraging the new technology will not be implemented: The new technology will not provide the anticipated value and it is highly likely that new workarounds will be added to the providers' daily work.

This becomes very challenging as the familiarity with the aging facility, processes, and technology does not always easily allow individuals to think beyond what they are used to in order to develop a map for the new facility design. Teams work very hard to visualize the new space, but in reality there are so many variables that this is often a daunting task for the teams. These variables include: size of the space, distance between spaces, storage locations, quantities stored, and specific locations of new technology.

In several instances, the aging inpatient facilities were replaced by more spacious rooms designed to accommodate the patients, their families, and multi-disciplinary caregiving teams. The new environments are often seen as much-improved healing spaces, and contain amazing new clinical and information technology. Without exception, the increased space and modern design are a welcomed relief.

The providers who experience this transition typically welcome it, but it is still change nonetheless. This change requires adaptation to a new environment, workflows, and processes. The education required to learn these new approaches often comes after a long shift and on top of a very demanding schedule.

Unintended Consequences of Space Redesign
Some unintended consequences to expanded space are the distance providers need to walk to take care of their patients and the increased diffi-culty of communicating in larger spaces. The basics that were so familiar in their previous environment are now very new, unfamiliar, and not as efficient. It has become more challenging for nurses to get through their new routines.

In the early phase of the change, there is a lot of excitement and hope for the future. This excitement and enthusiasm helps the multi-disciplinary team members work through the glitches in the processes. For example, walking the longer distances in a larger space is accepted at first. However, once this becomes more of a routine and patient volumes pick back up, the extra time required to reach the patient is perceived as an additional burden. After the newness wears off, providers report frustration with their new environments.

It typically takes some time to get settled into any new environment, and patient care settings are no exception. The duration of the transition depends on the magnitude of the change being undertaken. Following the process outlined in the following section should ease the transition to the new space.

Guidelines for Maximizing Workflow Design

In today's healthcare environment, there are numerous factors to consider when designing workflows within existing and/or new spaces. As the patient navigates through our continuum of care, they encounter numerous roles, equipment, spaces, and information systems. Each of these factors must be considered when designing or re-designing workflows. It is a very difficult assignment to design workflows given the intricacies of how each of these components interacts with the others. These six recommendations are guidelines we developed to maximize workflow design efforts.

Assemble a Multi-Disciplinary Workflow Design Team

Start with a multi-disciplinary team, including representation from each role that will work in the space. This often includes multiple roles such as hospitalists, primary care physicians, specialists, Advanced Practice Nurses, RNs, LPNs, therapists, and social workers.

Each party has a different view on including patients and their families in internal decision-making processes. However, we cannot assume that we know the patients' perspectives. Including them in workflow design can provide significant insights which can improve our workflow. On a few occasions, we've included patients in workflow design discussions and we've learned quite a bit from them. Their ideas are incorporated into our workflow and seem to provide improvements in our processes.

Roles that are often overlooked when designing workflows for existing and new space include team members from lab, radiology, pharmacy, house-keeping, transport, etc., who also work in the space to serve our patients. Additionally, there are a number of support roles, such as clinical engineering, facilities design, information services, patient access, revenue cycle, and finance that can provide significant expertise and insights into workflow design and impact the up- or downstream activities related to patient care. Peters and Waterman, authors of *In Search of Excellence* (2003), have been quoted as saying, "Leave no one out of the big picture. Involve everyone in everything of any consequence to all of you." While workflows are not the big picture, they are a critically important detail in the day of a caregiver. Involving each role in the creation of workflows can provide some significant benefits.

The multi-disciplinary team needs to include: (a) the patient—if the organization is comfortable with this; (b) each and every clinician role that will serve patients in that space; (c) any role which provides services to the patients in the space; and (d) roles that support caregivers with a variety of upstream and downstream activities.

Account for 100 Percent of the Roles, Equipment, and
Computer Systems Involved in the Workflow
This will be a very complex and tedious part of the process. However, accounting for as many details as possible will enhance workflow design. Start by listing the following:

1. All roles that serve the patient directly or indirectly in the space
2. Each piece of equipment that will be used to serve patients directly or indirectly in the space
3. Each computer software that will be used to serve patients directly or indirectly in the space

Follow the Patient Through the Space
It is very important to understand the current processes used to serve the patient. Physically walk through the space with the perspective of a patient, as well as of a provider, and account for the following:

1. Patient interactions with:

    a. Each role directly or indirectly serving the patient
    b. Each piece of equipment in the space
    c. Each computer program in the space

2. Each roles' interactions with:

    a. The patient
    b. Each piece of equipment in the space
    c. Each computer program in the space

This exercise will be very time consuming if done properly. Accounting for the above items will provide you with an excellent understanding of your current workflows.

Conduct Workflow Design Sessions in the Physical
Space or Simulate the Physical Space

Assemble your multi-disciplinary design team in the actual work space where the workflows will occur. Display your current workflows and begin to study the opportunities for improvement. Review the changes in space, equipment and/or computer systems that will be made to the existing environment, and determine any impacts on the current workflows.

Accounting for 100 percent of the roles, equipment, and computer systems involved in the workflow will provide tremendous challenges during this step in the process. However, there are potential benefits to properly account for most of the components that make up the workflows.

Set a goal to provide data and information to each role within the new workflow. Make it as easy as possible for the provider to complete their work. Avoid disruptions in workflow (e.g., a nurse leaving their workflow to retrieve a piece of equipment or to obtain some information). As much as possible, place the necessary equipment and data within the providers' workflow. This design principle should increase the providers' effectiveness, efficiency, and reduce their workload burden.

There have been numerous projects that did not properly account for one of the many factors listed above while designing workflows. The result is a component of overburden that we call workarounds. These workarounds often arise because the workflow process or space is not designed to account for 100 percent of the workflow components.

At that point, the caregivers have no choice but to create workarounds since they are directly interacting with the patients. These workarounds are often very creative because caregivers are very resourceful. However, if we properly include all components of the workflow during the design phase, we can eliminate many workarounds as they will be accounted for in the design rather than discovered afterwards. A proper workflow design should relieve the caregivers from having to create workarounds and should allow them to focus more of their energies on taking care of our patients.

When workflows are efficient and effective, the caregivers are freed up to focus on the work they have been trained to do—take care of patients. When workflows are inefficient and ineffective, caregivers' time, focus, and energy gets absorbed by wasteful processes or the creation of workarounds.

Conduct Physical Workflow Simulations Using Patient Actors for Each Role
A final step in the workflow design and creation is to simulate the workflow in the actual space where the workflow will occur. We often use patient actors who go through the workflow with the full team. An actor starts the journey through our workflow with each role interacting with them as if we were actually serving one of our patients.

The patient actor's role is used to view the workflow from the patient's perspective. I personally have served as a patient actor. Those who have also served as patient actors have provided feedback that it is quite an eye-opening experience. The feedback from these patient actors, as well as my personal experience as a patient actor, has indicated that even the smallest workflow item by any of the roles serving the patient may be magnified positively or negatively when viewed from the patient's perspective. Some things that do not seem important in a design session often times become very important from the patient's perspective.

Conducting this step is often overlooked, but may make the difference between good workflows and excellent workflows. Additionally, excellent workflows tend to reduce the burden on caregivers.

Adopt a Continuous Improvement Approach to Keeping Workflows Current
The healthcare environment is constantly changing due to advances in medicine, regulations, new equipment, technology, and computer software.

Once you have developed efficient and effective workflows, you will need to work very hard to keep them relevant and contemporary. With workflows, you typically learn a lot from actual use. The more you use them and socialize them, the more you tend to learn about opportunities for improvement.

As the environment around your workflow changes, you will find yourself in need of constantly adapting and adjusting your workflows. Therefore, deploy an approach to constantly measure, monitor, and improve your workflows to minimize the burden on your team.

This process improvement approach should be customer-focused, obtain direct input from those who use the workflows, and act upon feedback to continually improve your workflows. This will be an ongoing challenge, but may well prove to be worthwhile in improving the patient experience as well as reducing the burden on your team members.

Following the process outlined above will be very time-consuming. Many organizations do not invest the time up front to account for the patient and each role serving the patient either directly or indirectly. Some organizations do not understand the importance of this work.

Each organization will need to find the proper balance between the amount of time spent up front on workflow design efforts and the benefits of the time invested. Repeated cycles of workflow design are helpful, especially when simulated in the physical space or in a mock-up of the future, new physical space. Through these simulations, we can measure, learn about, and improve the effectiveness of the workflows, as well as obtain buy-in from each role that will need to serve our patients.

Obtaining buy-in from each role serving our patients is very important for the ongoing success in serving our patients. Getting the right multi-disciplinary team involved in workflow design will tend to improve the ownership of the workflows on a daily basis. Additionally, keeping the patient at the center of our workflow design processes, we need to account for each and every piece of equipment, as well as each and every computer system that will be used to provide care.

The rapidly changing healthcare industry is creating new pressures on our delivery system as well as those who work within this industry. The above process was documented as one potential way to reduce the burdens on caregivers by creating effective, efficient, repeatable, and reproducible workflows. Finally, it is recommended that a continuous improvement approach to monitoring and improving workflows be part of the fabric of every organization. This will be one step to monitor the burden placed on caregivers by an ever-changing healthcare environment.

Information Technology Considerations

Meaningful use has created tremendous pressures to automate the care delivery processes and is also introducing requirements to electronically communicate with patients. Meaningful use is using certified electronic health record technology to:

- Improve quality, safety, efficiency, and reduce health disparities
- Engage patients and family
- Improve care coordination, population, and public health
- Maintain privacy and security of patient health information

Ultimately, it is hoped that the meaningful use compliance will result in:

- Better clinical outcomes
- Improved population health outcomes
- Increased transparency and efficiency
- Empowered individuals
- More robust research data on health systems

Meaningful use sets specific objectives that eligible professionals (EPs) and hospitals must achieve to qualify for Centers for Medicare and Medicaid Services (CMS) Incentive Programs (Centers for Medicare and Medicaid, 2015).

The Meaningful Use program has also increased the deployment of mobile equipment such as laptops, smartphones, tablets, and numerous other devices to support the providers' experiences. As clinical and information technology continues to advance, more and more clinical equipment and information technology is introduced into our aging facilities. Multidisciplinary teams must work extremely hard to find adequate storage space for the new devices and technology in aging facilities. For example, it frequently becomes difficult to find space to store and/or re-charge the batteries in some of the new mobile equipment.

As we add equipment and technology to the model, it becomes increasingly multifaceted, so much so that we removed the communication lines so that the model would still be legible. However, the model has become very cluttered, indicating the complexity of the healthcare system (see Figure 4).

The patient is still at the center, but the complexity of the model that patients and providers navigate becomes very challenging.

The diagram illustrates equipment and technology as three small circles for each role. In health care today, individuals in each role typically have more pieces of equipment or information technology components to deal with than is illustrated here. There can be anywhere from two to twenty medical devices in a patient room and the provider may need to access one to ten computer systems to provide care to a patient. As our simple diagram shows, the patient remains right in the middle of the complex interactions of roles, communication, equipment, and technology.

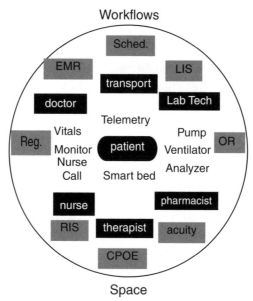

FIGURE 4. **Complexity of Interactions with the Patient**

As a result, it becomes increasingly difficult to serve the needs of the patient in efficient and effective ways. To ensure we make our best attempt to minimize the burden of this complexity, we need to account for each role, piece of equipment, and computer system in workflow design as described earlier in this chapter.

Our patients and each associated role want the processes to be simple and clear. They also want things to work each and every time. We need to use this as a design principle in any new workflow development process.

Information technology solutions should strive to capture the data accurately at the point of creation and distribute that data to each role as necessary. The delivery of this data to each role should be incorporated directly into the respective workflows. Each role should not be required to break out of their natural work flow to seek out the needed data.

However, the complexities of the patient, healthcare providers, healthcare operations, space, equipment, and technology are significant. It is understandable why each component has been architected separately in many instances. The complexity of this model requires a substantial comparison of current state and future state. This task can seem daunting for teams of people who are operating at maximum capacity within this complexity. They are working hard to meet day-to-day demands and typically do not have adequate time to develop the necessary analysis to introduce new equipment and information technology.

Information Overload and Organizational Architecture: Countering the Complexity

As represented in this chapter's simple model, the complexities of the healthcare industry are significant and can be overwhelming. Steven J. Spear (2009) described the challenges each complex organization faces as follows:

> ... they produce complex products or provide complex services, requiring many varied forms of skill and expertise ... their "systems of work" ... are correspondingly complex ... the more numerous and varied the people, machines and materials, the more ways they can interact ... Eventually, so much is connected to so much else that the system becomes "unknowable."

The healthcare industry certainly has become a highly complex industry. The simple model used in this chapter demonstrates the complexity of the environment. In reality, the healthcare environment is much more complex than this simple model was able to demonstrate.

The workflow design considerations section above (see page 43) was intended to provide some suggestions to consider for countering this complexity. We have included below some additional considerations as new space and/or workflow are being designed and developed:

1. Top Three Principles Guiding Understanding and Application

    a. Keep the patient at the center of the space and workflow design

    b. Account for each role in the healthcare environment

    c. Adopt a continuous improvement approach to workflows

2. Tips and Tools for Applying High Reliability Practices

    a. Have the people interacting directly with the patient (e.g., sharp end) develop the architecture for the space and workflow

    b. Establish a change governance process to allocate resources, remove barriers, empower change teams, and champion the organizational change

    c. Health care organizations should spend most of their time on the three to five things that have the greatest value to the patient

3. Actionable Tactics for Consideration
   a. Create a matrix of role-to-role interactions
   b. Document how each role will interact with the patient
   c. Document how each role will utilize each
      i. Piece of equipment
      ii. Computer system

As the healthcare environment becomes more and more complex, the ability to adapt to the complexity has become more important. Transformation of healthcare will require that complex changes are made to address complex needs, and space is one of those. Identifying a comprehensive approach that will work in your organization will be challenging. This chapter is intended to offer, for your consideration, some approaches that have worked in certain environments to counter the complexity and to support you in your very important work—serving your patients.

References

Center for Medicare and Medicaid. (2014). 2014 definition stage 1 of meaningful use. Retrieved from www.cms.gov/Regulations-and-Guidance/Legislation/EHRIncentivePrograms/Meaningful_Use.html

Churchill, W. (1941). You do your worst—And we will do our best. Retrieved from http://www.winstonchurchill.org/resources/speeches/1941-1945-war-leader

Peters, T. & Waterman, R. (2003). *In search of excellence*. New York, NY: Collins Publishing.

Spear, S. (2009). *The high-velocity edge*. New York, NY: McGraw-Hill.

Weick, K. E., & Sutcliffe, K. M. (2001). *Managing the unexpected*. San Francisco, CA: Jossey-Bass.

4

Leadership in a Complex World

Jason H. Gilbert, BSN, MBA and
Marion E. Broome, PhD, RN, FAAN

Case Study: Carrie Tackles the Acuity Implementation

Carrie returns to her office from the town hall meeting, sits at her desk, and puts her head into her hands. Carrie is the Operations Director for Nursing who has been given the responsibility of implementing a new software platform to measure nursing acuity for the facility. Although the clinical departments do not report to her directly, she is confident in her ability to implement it. During the town hall meeting, the project took a turn for the worse and now seems impossible. Because budgets are tight, the project has great implications for increasing nursing efficiency and accurately capturing workload. The organization has just faced a series of budget reductions, and when Carrie asked for clinical representation for the steering team from her Director colleagues, she was told that the units cannot afford any more time off of the unit. Not wanting to cause any discord, Carrie felt that she would be able to come up with the system design and implementation plan by herself. After meeting with several key stakeholders, she confidently started working on the implementation plan.

Carrie spends the next weeks analyzing benchmarking data, labor standards, productivity data, billing information, and financial performance data for each area. She does her homework and comes up with an extremely detailed design and implementation plan that she is certain is the right course. She has poured over the details, has a data point to back every decision, and is very confident in her plan. She gives regular updates on her progress to her Director colleagues and to her boss. Everything is going well, and she is ahead of schedule. Carrie's boss seems pleased with her progress and asks her to give a presentation at the nursing town hall as a way to build excitement and communicate the implementation plan.

Carrie gives a flawless presentation. She makes sure that all of the information is offered, graphs with supportive data are included, and the very detailed implementation plan is presented. She smiles as she finishes the presentation, looking out over the crowd. Carrie asks, "What questions do you have?", assuming that there would be none since the plan and presentation are rock-solid. One hand is raised in the back of the room.

"I don't understand a thing you just said. You talked about the benefits of this system, but I don't believe you! I heard this is a way for you to cut staffing. How do you expect us to take care of more patients? No one asked our opinion."

The presentation deteriorates from there. Several angry comments are made by staff members and Nurse Managers. Carrie is surprised to learn that half of the Nurse Managers have not even heard of the project. Many are upset about the timeframe given to other projects, and others give reasons that this plan cannot possibly work for their area. Carrie attempts to bring the group back around to no avail. No matter what she says, she is not able to change the mood in the room. Finally her boss steps in and states that the plan will be revised based on the feedback provided and more information will be forthcoming.

Carrie sits at her desk after the meeting and thinks about what went wrong. Why is this so hard? She knows that she articulated clearly and worked out so many details that all anyone had to do was follow the plan. After all, she has been always been told she is an excellent communicator and is able to understand the big picture. Why, then, did she feel that she was eaten alive in the town hall meeting today as she presented the implementation plan?

Carrie opens an email from her boss asking for her to meet tomorrow to discuss revising the implementation plan for the acuity system. What happened? How could she recover from this? What is she going to tell her boss? Carrie pulls out a blank piece of paper and begins to reflect on what could have possibly gone wrong.

The Changing Face of Leadership in a Complex World

The nature of leadership in modern healthcare organizations has changed dramatically in the past decades as free standing hospitals and other healthcare facilities have reorganized and merged into large complex interconnected networks and systems. The complexity of these "living" systems will continue to evolve and change as the implementation of the Affordable Care Act of 2010 brings the greatest changes to the American healthcare system since the advent of Medicare and Medicaid services in 1965 (The Institute of Medicine at the National Academies, 2010). Economic and social pressures for performance in patient satisfaction, quality, and financial performance metrics will undoubtedly increase the complexity of leadership in modern healthcare organizations. It is predicted that by the year 2020 up to one out of three hospitals will either reorganize into a different structure or close in response to the massive changes required for viability (Everett & Sitterding, 2013; Fleece & Houle, 2011).

How is the nature of leadership changing? Traditional models of leadership are shifting from top-down approaches to incorporate principles of manager as coach, mentor, advisor, facilitator, and teacher within the complex team (Heller et al., 2004). Many healthcare organizations began during the industrial era in the U.S. and adopted the assembly line type design in which the leadership style was hierarchical and focused on a top-down solution-oriented approach (Lindberg, Nash, & Lindberg, 2008; Zimmerman, Lindberg, & Plsek, 2001). This has led to the separation of disciplines and governance into distinct entities within hospitals. Managers were once viewed as experts who were focused on command and control of employees in order to achieve organizational goals.

While this approach may have traditionally worked in environments focused solely on the production of physical products, this approach has failed as information exchange and technology have shifted the economic model to focus on knowledge work (Uhl-Bien, Marion, & McKelvey, 2007; Zimmerman et al., 2001). Nurses and other healthcare professionals are knowledge workers who must synthesize information learned through formal education and experience in the delivery of safe and effective care

(Porter-O'Grady, 2003). Knowledge workers require different leadership styles in their managers than traditional workers. Yet, many of the hierarchical models of leadership and distinct role definitions and structures still exist today, causing difficulty in navigating and leading change in healthcare systems. The modern healthcare organization may be thought of as a "living system" in which interconnected parts react to inputs and then interact as outcomes are produced.

Not only has the economic shift from the industrial era to the knowledge era changed the nature of leadership, but evolution of social interactions has shifted the ability to enact command and control. Technological advances and access to information have shifted the power differentials in traditional leadership models (Kellerman, 2012). Prior to the ubiquity of social media, opinions and ideas were largely left to the identified experts in the field. Now ordinary people are able to reach and influence a larger arena through the use of technology such as Facebook, Twitter, LinkedIn, and various blogs and websites. This has greatly influenced effective thought and behavior of followers and has shifted the paradigm away from the leader as the all-knowing, all-powerful expert. Access to information and the ability to connect with a large network has created the expectation of "participative democracy," in which followers expect to have a voice in a collective decision-making process (Kellerman, 2012). One only needs to turn on the television to see this played out through competition-based television programming in which public votes decide the outcome.

A shift in economic drivers, reorganization into large systems, increased governmental regulations, technological advances making information readily accessible, and a shift in the social contracts between leaders and followers have all made leadership more difficult in modern healthcare organizations. It is difficult—if not impossible—to find leaders with all of the required knowledge, skills, and experience necessary to successfully navigate large complex organizations through uncharted territory (Carmeli & Tishler, 2004a; Carmeli & Tishler, 2004b; Kor & Mesko, 2013). The interaction and relationships between individuals in a system will become more important as healthcare systems continue to evolve. Leaders who can adapt to this new model of leadership based on influence rather than authority, who can be resilient, who can embrace change and unpredictable outcomes, and who can effectively take risks and learn from mistakes are those who will likely be successful in the future.

Complex Adaptive Systems Theory

Modern healthcare organizations have evolved into what may be defined as a complex adaptive system (CAS). Rooted in complexity science, CAS theory is especially useful in explaining the sometimes unpredictable outcomes that emerge from interactions of individual parts and groups in relationships seen in biology, economics, and the social sciences. A CAS is a collection of individual agents that may interact in an unpredictable manner in order to maximize some measure of quality or fitness (Tan, Wen, & Awad, 2005). These interconnected and diverse agents may have connections with other entities that interact and co-evolve as information and resources are shared (Lindberg et al., 2008). Within a CAS, individuals and groups act through their own schema, historical context, and organizational view in order to produce an outcome (Zimmerman et al., 2001). Since the interactions and relationships between individuals in a CAS is a factor that precipitates co-evolution, often times the connections are viewed as more important than the individuals within the system (Burns, 2001). Characteristics of a CAS may be found in Table 2 (Alaa & Fitzgerald, 2013; Burns, 2001; Lindberg et al., 2008; Metcalf & Benn, 2012; Tan et al., 2005; Zimmerman et al., 2001).

A principle central to CAS theory is that of dwelling at the edge of chaos to maximize innovation. In an industrial model comprised only of machines, outcomes can be controlled through programming machines to act in a predictable manner (Waltuck, 2012). This does not hold true in a CAS, which thrives on the unpredictable nature of a chaotic environment as individuals interact and co-evolve (Burns, 2001). This is not to say that there is not a time and place for a mechanistic view in health care, such as in highly technical and evidence-based procedures in which predictable outcomes are necessary, but organizations and leaders who attempt to control every aspect of the environment often fail to harness outcomes through innovation and evolution of processes (Burns, 2001).

Chaos is not completely random, but is largely unpredictable because of the nature of human interactions in organizations. Healthcare systems require a wide variance in knowledge and skills of the individual agents interacting in many different ways (Burns, 2001; Tan et al., 2005). The key to allowing the organization to thrive at the edge of chaos is the flow of information and communication in the organization (Lindberg et al., 2008; Lindberg & Schneider, 2012; Zimmerman et al., 2001). If there is not enough information, there may be too much control and little creativity. If there is too much, there may be total chaos. The key to effective leadership

TABLE 2. **Complex Adaptive System Characteristics**

Characteristic	Description
Diversity	Diverse individuals and groups within the CAS having diverse opinions, thoughts, and information of the system. The more diverse, the more the overall health of the system is improved as innovation and creativity is enhanced.
Self-organization	Connections and relationships formed among different agents and systems embedded in the CAS. The results emerge through self-organization and through the interactions between individuals and groups rather than through a centrally defined organization.
Embeddedness	Separate complex systems are embedded within a larger CAS. A nurse may work within a dialysis center in a large medical center that is embedded within a large healthcare system. These embedded parts co-evolve as changes in one part affect the others.
Distributed Control	Control does not come from a central command location. Control is distributed throughout the system to allow for flexibility and adaptability as the interconnected parts evolve.
Nonlinear Dynamics and Emergence	Outcomes may not correlate well with the size of the input. A large effort to change may not move the system while a small change effort may have large scale effects. The dynamics are difficult to predict. Patterns of outcomes emerge as a result of interactions, history, learning, and adaptation within the system.
Adaptable	Change occurs as a result of the interaction of the individual agents and groups in the system. Dynamic tension from the environment, organizational norms, social interactions, and resource allocation create the impetus that changes and adapts in response to pressure.
Order and Disorder Exist Simultaneously	Some patterns and outcomes may be well organized and predictable, while others may be volatile or chaotic as interactions occur.

in this case is to find the right balance of information flow to and from those involved in various initiatives, as well as among all those individuals.

The Evolving Role of Nurse Leaders in Complex Systems

If a CAS is self-organizing, and it is ideal to have a distributed control to optimize outcomes, then what is the role of the nurse leader in the organization? Should the nurse leader sit back and let the living system evolve, self-organize, and emerge in response to dynamic tensions? The answer to this question is no, but the ideals for effective leadership have evolved and will continue to do so given the environmental pressures already mentioned. The role of the leader in a CAS should be largely interpretive in nature and can be the element that improves the adaptability and sustainability of the organization (Metcalf & Benn, 2012; Metcalf & Benn 2013). Leaders in these complex environments must be able to see the big picture and have an understanding of how the system interacts, while at the same time be able to 'zoom in' when necessary to view the needs of those involved in the work of the organization (Kanter, 2011).

In traditional models of leadership, managers were viewed as the principle agent of change through planning, direction, and control. In the CAS, a leader may not always be viewed as the principle change agent, but more often as the agent that influences the conditions in which change is produced. Leadership competencies in the CAS include assessment and understanding of the complexity of the system, communication, complex problem solving, trial and error, acceptance of ambiguity and unknown results, harnessing the creativity and potential of individuals, and the ability to deal with conflict and tension in the system (Lichtenstein et al., 2006; Lindberg et al., 2008; Metcalf & Benn, 2013; Tan et al., 2005; Zimmerman et al., 2001).

This is not to say that command and control styles of leadership need be abandoned completely. Effectiveness of leadership style is context dependent and will rest on the organization, the environment, or the immediate situation (Seiler & Pfister, 2009). A balance of leadership styles is necessary dependent on the situational context. It is important for nurse leaders to balance when a directive style is warranted and when decentralized control is a better approach.

Effective nurse leaders are therefore challenged to adapt to new models of thinking and evolving styles of leadership. No leader, however strong, could possibly possess all knowledge, skills, and experience necessary to lead complex organizations even in smaller organizational units such as patient care units or departments of similar units (Carmeli & Tishler, 2004a). Nurse leaders must now become more of a mentor, coach, teacher, facilitator, and advisor (Heller et al., 2004). Nurse leaders must strive to create context and meaning for individuals in an organization, and be highly adept at translating and communicating within the large organization.

Learning to Let Go of Control

Leadership behavior can emerge at any level of a CAS through self-organizing behavior in reaction to an event (Lichtenstein et al., 2006; Seiler & Pfister, 2009; Zimmerman et al., 2001). Many different conceptual models have outlined the importance of embracing leadership at all levels and the importance to healthcare outcomes. In her acclaimed book *High Performance Healthcare*, Jody Gittell (2009) notes that high-performing teams built on mutual respect, shared goals, and shared knowledge within which communication is frequent, timely, accurate, and problem solving in nature produce better outcomes. Gittell further notes that a decentralized model of leadership and breaking down functional silos within organizations are game changers in terms of enhanced performance.

The American Nurses Credentialing Center (ANCC) Magnet Designation is considered the gold standard for recognition of organizations employing nurses in terms of nursing work environments and quality of nursing care outcomes (Broom & Tilbury, 2007; McHugh et al., 2013). One of the components of the Magnet Model has been transformational leadership, in which organizations must demonstrate the participation of the direct care nurse in organizational decision making (American Nurses Credentialing Center, 2014). This model demonstrates the importance of decentralized locus of control for achieving organizational outcomes.

Why, then, is learning to give up control so difficult for nurse leaders? The short answer: It is risky. Many healthcare organizations still hold onto very traditional values and styles of leadership. In organizations where functional silos and hierarchical management models exist, it will be more difficult for the nurse leader to allow for self-organizing behavior of the nursing workforce and create an environment where innovation thrives. The organizational context and culture may limit the ability of the nurse leader to enact this evolved model of leadership successfully (Seiler & Pfister, 2009), and nurse leaders must advocate for involvement of the front-line staff. The nurse leader will need to be courageous and embrace the notion that outcomes may not always be what were planned. Lessening personal control and empowering others to act may be risky, but it can also be a great benefit to the leader through the creation of collaborative relationships that enhance outcomes (Kouzes & Posner, 2012).

Being Comfortable with Life on the Edge

Anyone who stands on the rim of the Grand Canyon or at the edge of a tall building may have the feeling of sweaty palms, increased heart rate, vertigo, or the fear that they are going to tumble to their certain demise. Letting go of control and allowing for the organization to live at the edge of chaos can feel very similar. The right conditions must exist in order for this to happen: you must have the right amount of information flow, diversity, connection among individuals, and level of dynamic tension (Zimmerman et al., 2001). If too few of these elements exist, there is no reason for change, and processes remain stagnant and mechanistic; too many of any of these elements, and there is complete disorder and the systems could collapse (Tan et al., 2005; Waltuck, 2012).

How, then, does a nurse leader become comfortable allowing for this edge-of-collapse perspective? It begins with the recruitment and retention of a diverse and talented workforce and facilitating connections between individuals and teams within the system. Facilitating connection between key stakeholders and helping them understand how they fit within the larger system is important. The nurse leader must understand the network of connections, use the connections to affect outcomes, and create new connections in order to be successful. Translating information in a meaningful way to teams without a large data dump is also helpful in assisting others to assimilate meaning. That is, the nurse leader must be wary of just providing numbers, performance charts, and metrics without some interpretation of the meaning within the context of that unit. Finally, many times nurse leaders believe that they need to take on all of the tension that the team feels. Without the team feeling some of the strain and participating in the decision, the nurse leader has little hope of motivating others to change. Many organizational changes are doomed to fail in the very beginning by neglecting to establish a sense of urgency in realistic terms (Kotter, 2007).

It takes practice to identify the right balance of information, diversity, connection, and tension to keep the team at the edge of chaos. Nurse leaders should evaluate the risks and benefits before embarking on a major change that could have dire consequences to patients. This is also not to be confused with a laissez-faire style of management in which the leader leaves the team completely alone to fend for themselves. Small tests of change can be done with this in order to gauge both team and organizational readiness for life at the edge of chaos.

Get Out of the Data Trap

As nurse leaders have an imperative to assist others in assimilating meaning in their work, one of the slippery slopes is the amount of data and metrics that are produced in healthcare organizations. Given the advances in information technology and the imperative to report a multitude of data points to various regulatory, governmental, and benchmarking bodies, there is never a lack of information available on any topic in the organization. So much information is produced by organizations that it far surpasses the human ability to process it all in a meaningful way (Farhoomand & Drury, 2002).

Individuals vary in their capacity to receive and process information, and there is a threshold in which information receipt is only valuable up to the individual's capacity to process and handle information (Oldroyd & Morris, 2012). After this threshold, information overload sets in and performance sharply declines, causing poor decision-making and lower productivity (Farhoomand & Drury, 2002; Oldroyd & Morris, 2012). The phenomenon of constantly living in a state of information overload causes what may be defined as "continuous partial attention," in which individuals are unable to fully give full cognitive attention to a task given the multiple and simultaneous demands caused by information and technology (Stone, 2007).

Contributing factors to information overload for clinicians may include failure to process data, processing data incorrectly, a delay in processing, acceptance of low quality data, and giving up on the search for other information (Clarke et al., 2013). It is further noted that the way in which the information is presented, the context in which it is presented, and the available amount of time the individual has to work with the information also lead to information overload (Hall & Walton, 2004). Strategies to overcome the effects of information overload include reducing the number of extraneous metrics and asking clinicians what information is important to measure as an outcome (Clarke et al., 2013).

Nurse leaders are in a unique position to access the multitude of information and data that exists in the organization. Often leaders make the mistake of displaying metric after metric with the hope that this will equate with understanding or agreement with the plan of action. The rationale to support this behavior is often, "If people just see the numbers, they will naturally understand why things must change and be rallied to action." Although this strategy may work with a few individuals, this is, overall, a dangerous trap that may actually undermine the success of the project. Nurse leaders must first clearly define and communicate the goal or outcome, choose the metrics that really matter in conjunction with those who will carry out the project, remove resource constraints, synthesize, simplify, and translate meaningful data to the teams that they lead.

The Key to Unlocking Unlimited Potential: Communication

The only tool that a leader has to successfully enact change is communication. As simplistic as this statement sounds, it can be very complex. It can be even more difficult to communicate to a wide number of people working on different shifts every day of the week. Given that the economic drivers of health care have changed, the nature of leadership has evolved, and the advanced expectation of followers has shifted to including them as participants, nurse leaders must think differently about the way they communicate. It is noted that many leaders fail by engaging in either the wrong types of communication or unproductive communication (Ford & Ford, 2009).

In the mechanistic era, carrot and stick communication was used to maintain equilibrium and control in repetitive environments (Pink, 2011). Certainly there is a place for this in the modern organization, but communicating only tasks and consequences will stifle innovation and lead to a disengaged workforce. Different forms of communication may be employed in order to improve outcomes and innovation. Transformational leadership styles employed in organizations have been shown to produce better outcomes through the development of individuals to their full potential (Northouse, 2013). Transformational communication includes idealized influence (in which the leader is a strong role model to followers), inspirational motivation (in which leaders communicate high expectations and vision), intellectual stimulation (in which leaders stimulate creativity and innovation), and individualized consideration (in which the leader provides a supportive environment where the voice of the follower is heard) (Northouse, 2013).

So how does this work in practice? Often nurse leaders spend too much time planning and spelling out all of the details of a change in the hopes that if the followers fully understand the plan, there will not be a problem. Often times the nurse leader must have courage to communicate a vision that is good enough, meaning that not every detail needs to be decided up front; the adaptive system will work out some of the details as the initiative progresses (Zimmerman et al., 2001). Leaders need to communicate clearly what the outcome needs to be and why it is important, but not necessarily how each detail must be completed. If a rationale for the importance of a task is communicated, and individuals are given the autonomy to complete a task their own way when possible, the result is likely to be an engaged and motivated workforce (Pink, 2011).

Leaders may amplify the rate of organizational change and the success of initiatives through communication. Leaders who promote interactive communication in which ideas are shared, learning is a goal, and individuals are motivated to stretch to their full potential will realize that individuals will take initiative to make meaningful contributions (Kouzes & Posner, 2012). In order for this to occur, the nurse leader must create an environment in which individuals feel safe from fear of retribution. This environment of safety must be communicated in all forms, including the behaviors of the leader. As a state of disequilibrium occurs in a system, the nurse leader may influence emergence of improved outcomes by allowing for experiments in which teams have permission to try new ideas and learn from mistakes, encouraging rich interactions in which teams are given time and space to interact and forge working relationships, and supporting collective action through allowing for and celebrating teams who collectively work to solve organizational issues (Lichtenstein & Plowman, 2009).

Resistance to change is a phenomenon on which there are volumes of literature written. Communications are planned around resistance, leaders cringe when dissenting opinions are voiced in organizations, and hours are wasted around planning strategies to minimize and combat resistance. When presented with a change, people attempt to make sense and gather meaning from the communication presented (Ford, Ford, & D'Amelio, 2008). Resistance may be viewed as an important feedback mechanism that gives important cues to the leader on how the system is interacting or changes that may be necessary in the communication pattern. Resistance often occurs as a result of a lack of agreement, a violation of trust, or communication issues such as a poor call to action, failure to legitimize change, or misrepresentation of the impact of the initiative (Ford et al., 2008). The counter-offers and feedback provided when encountering perceived resistance may be extremely valuable in execution of the initiative. Understanding the gossip, rumors, and informal relationships that exist in an organization may assist the leader in predicting the behavior of others (Zimmerman et al., 2001).

Reflection and Planning
The world of nursing practice within complex institutions requires leaders, both in formal and less formal positions, to lead through engagement of others. By engaging with others one can better assess all aspects of any problem affecting the environment in which safe and high-quality care must be delivered and experienced by patients. Once one obtains from

others their perspectives on an issue, it is time to turn inward and assess one's own perspective and how one is dealing with a situation. The ability to zoom in and zoom out when faced with a challenge (Kanter, 2011) in the workplace often determines the effectiveness of a leader in addressing complicated issues.

Critical reflection on important incidents in which what one expected to happen doesn't happen is an opportunity for learning. Yet, the concept of learning from mistakes often has a negative connotation. In fact, the fast-paced environments of health care in which leaders work often seem chaotic and one that leaves little time for reflective thinking. Additionally, in some workplaces, there sometimes appears to be a zero tolerance for mistakes or errors, even when they don't directly affect patients. Finally, the emotions that often accompany any 'failed' initiative can be overwhelming, especially for individuals who are organized, strategic, and have high expectations for themselves.

One of the most challenging skills for an emerging leader to learn is the art of self-reflection. Self-reflection is defined as the ability to learn to be aware of one's actions, how they affect others, and how to envision how one might behave differently when engaging with others (Horton-Deutsch, 2013). Any organization that is successful in negotiating the constant change that is essential to survival supports individuals who can learn from their mistakes and who are encouraged by mentors to take time to self-reflect on their behavior and actions and how those actions impacted the situation. These are individuals who, when Plan A is not successful in moving things forward, will not just develop a Plan B on the spot but have actually already thought the plan through in terms of implementation. This kind of planning entails anticipating what can go wrong before the initiative is even implemented; having strategies lined up to address potential barriers or pitfalls helps to ensure effective execution. Asking oneself several questions in the planning phase of an initiative will promote developing multiple scenarios when one is planning an initiative (see Sidebar 1).

This will require that a leader engage with those who will be involved in the execution to gain their assessments about what might happen as things evolve, then give serious consideration to incorporating their assessments and suggestions in any execution plan. A leader who is humble enough to do this will gain the respect of those they work with and model the kind of leadership behaviors that facilitate a successful execution of plans (Tjan, 2012).

Sidebar 1—Scenarios to Guide Planning

The following questions should be considered in the pre-planning phase of an implementation to account for all possible challenges that may be encountered:

- Will this change require providers on a unit (in a department) to change the way they deliver care now?
- If so, what kinds of support will we have to provide for them to change the processes they use now?
- Who should we talk with or observe before we develop the implementation plan?
- What if the providers refuse to change the processes?
- Who in that department can help us to understand what is working well and what isn't while the initiative evolves?
- What benefits can the providers expect after changing their processes?

Adapting and Building Resiliency

Adapting to changing conditions is easiest when one has some influence over the situation. By engaging in reflective thinking before and after an initiative is implemented, one can think through many what-ifs—some of which may be more plausible, less costly, more efficient, or more effective—as well as what actually happened. After several situations in which one is able to pair these what-ifs with the corresponding actions, one becomes more confident and resilient when the next initiative comes along.

Resiliency is defined as "the developable capacity to rebound or bounce back from adversity, conflict, and failure or even positive events, progress and increased responsibility" (Luthans, 2002, p. 702). Many individuals, when faced with increased responsibility that doesn't result in outcomes they expect, can become disappointed and even resentful. Resilient leaders, upon constructive self-reflection, are able to see challenge as an opportunity. They are able to reconstruct how they interact with others or implement certain projects, and can see themselves as being able to change their behavior in a way that will increase their effectiveness. This in turn fosters an emerging leader's willingness to maintain hope and optimism (Youssef & Luthans, 2007) and take calculated risks when planning initiatives.

Conclusion: Advice for Carrie and the Acuity Tool Implementation

What could Carrie have done differently in her approach to the acuity system implementation? She may have done too much planning independently and did not seek the input of those who would be carrying out the work. Although she did seek out the opinion and input of her director colleagues and give them regular updates, she did not negotiate more resources in terms of staffing for the project. Carrie may have been more successful in gaining support from the directors if she had stressed the importance of staff input and involvement in this clinical initiative, made sessions focused, and limited presentation time. Although Carrie did a great deal of planning, she may have tried to plan too many aspects of the project in the hopes that the organization would not feel the strain of implementation. She thought that she could anticipate every challenge independently, and may have created more negative resistance in reaction to a well-orchestrated plan. Carrie may have overwhelmed the group further with excessive data to the point of cognitive overload. Carrie's presentation may have been more effective had she better communicated the overall goals and focused on a few metrics rather than attempting to solve every issue in the project up front.

Despite these issues, there are several actions that Carrie did well. The first was the self-reflection which she started to engage in at the end of the case. She did engage in a great deal of planning, and the implementation plan is likely not a complete loss. She will need to work closely with different agents embedded in the system to receive feedback on parts of the plan that may work, effectively identify anticipated barriers, and engage others in the process. Certainly Carrie is frustrated that the plan was not accepted as is by the individuals in the system, but these plans rarely are. Carrie can view the reactions and comments as feedback cues for where her plan may need work rather than labeling them simply as resistance. Whether or not Carrie realizes it, her communication and the reaction experienced by her audience may have caused a state of disequilibrium that could viably be harnessed in order to effectively implement the acuity system. The fact that Carrie is reflecting at the end of the case on what may have gone wrong is an important first step. Engaging in self-reflection and taking accountability for the misjudgments she made will enable her to regroup and adapt based on the feedback from the system. If Carrie can admit her mistakes, ask for assistance of the team, and create an environment in which others will engage in the process, she will be able to correct the course of the project. Certainly there are many pitfalls and unforeseen problems that a nurse leader must adapt to during any initiative. Sidebar 2 gives a list of useful questions to aid in self-reflection before tackling a change initiative.

Leadership in modern complex systems is indeed very challenging and takes a great deal of courage. Table 3 outlines key messages established in this chapter.

Although the concepts presented in this chapter seem simplistic, they are very difficult to enact and practice in environments with competing priorities, limited budgets, high-stakes outcomes, complex reporting structures, challenging organizational politics, and high pressure for performance. Nurse leaders must change the traditional views of leadership and move toward more influential, transformational styles of leadership to meet the challenges ahead. Those who are able to adapt to unknown futures in complex environments will certainly be empowered to lead engaged teams who will innovate healthcare delivery for future generations.

Sidebar 2—Self-Reflection on Project Planning and Implementation

- What is the overall goal of this project? What is absolutely necessary to have? What is nice to have? What is negotiable?
- What style do I feel most comfortable with when leading a project? Do I plan everything out and then seek input, or seek input on goals and processes first?
- Who needs to be involved in this project? How do I communicate with others who need to know what is being planned? What is being implemented?
- What metrics will be used? How will they be measured and communicated? Do I have too many measures?
- When I do seek input, do I incorporate it or find reasons the suggestion won't work?
- What barriers to implementation are anticipated? How can I remove those? Who can I collaborate with to identify and remove barriers?
- If someone is highly critical when providing feedback how do/will I respond to them?
- Have I created a safe environment in which diverse views are heard and incorporated if necessary?
- How do I share the changes I have made?
- If a project is successful, how do I credit the work of others? What specific strategies do I use? How can I support collective action of the teams?

TABLE 3. **Key Messages**

The nature of leadership is evolving	Economic models have shifted from industrial era to knowledge era. Expectations of leaders have shifted through societal changes and social media. Leaders must adapt to lead through participative influence rather than command and control traits. Learning to let go of centralized control is necessary for success.
Healthcare organizations are evolving into complex adaptive systems	Most healthcare organizations are evolving into large, complex networks of interconnected agents that may react in an unpredictable manner. Leaders may influence conditions in which innovation and self-organization is optimized through recognizing and creating connections between teams and individuals.
Diversity will drive outcomes	Recruitment and retention of a talented, diverse workforce with divergent views will enhance the quality of outcomes within systems.
Too much data can be overwhelming	Rather than getting confused by too much data, pick a few key metrics that are the most important to track for quality improvement. Translating data in a meaningful way is essential for team success.
Communication is everything	Mastering communication in all forms is essential for the leader's ability to influence others. Through words, actions, and behaviors, leaders may inspire others to act and create safe environments for participation.
Reflection and planning help leaders face challenging situations	Self-reflection and thoughtful planning give the leader the ability to learn from mistakes and anticipate challenges successfully.
Adaptation and resiliency are essential characteristics of leaders	The future is uncertain and the ability to adapt to unforeseen challenges and develop resiliency is an opportunity for professional growth and success.

References

Alaa, G., & Fitzgerald, G. (2013). Re-conceptualizing agile information systems development using complex adaptive systems theory. *Emergence: Complexity & Organization, 15*(3), 1–23.

Broom, C., & Tilbury, M. S. (2007). Magnet status: A journey, not a destination. *Journal of Nursing Care Quality, 22*(2), 113–118.

Burns, J. P. (2001). Complexity science and leadership in healthcare. *Journal of Nursing Administration, 31*(10), 474–482.

Carmeli, A., & Tishler, A. (2004a). The relationships between intangible organizational elements and organizational performance. *Strategic Management Journal, 25*(13), 1257–1278. doi: 10.1002/smj.428

Carmeli, A., & Tishler, A. (2004b). Resources, capabilities, and the performance of industrial firms: A multivariate analysis. *Managerial and Decision Economics, 25*(6/7), 299–315. doi: 10.1002/mde.1192

Clarke, M. A., Belden, J. L., Koopman, R. J., Steege, L. M., Moore, J. L., Canfield, S. M., & Kim, M. S. (2013). Information needs and information-seeking behaviour analysis of primary care physicians and nurses: A literature review. *Health Information & Libraries Journal, 30*(3), 178–190. doi: 10.1111/hir.12036

Everett, L. Q., & Sitterding, M. C. (2013). Building a culture of innovation by maximizing the role of the RN. *Nursing Administration Quarterly, 37*(3), 194–202. doi: 10.1097/NAQ.0b013e318295ed7f

Farhoomand, A. F., & Drury, D. H. (2002). Managerial information overload. *Communications of the ACM, 45*(10), 127–131.

Fleece, J., & Houle, D. (2011). *New health age: The future of health care in America.* Naperville, IL: Sourcebooks, Inc.

Ford, J. D., & Ford, L. W. (2009). *The four conversations: Daily communication that gets results.* San Francisco, CA: Berrett-Koehler Publishers.

Ford, J. D., Ford, L. W., & D'Amelio, A. (2008). Resistance to change: The rest of the story. *Academy of Management Review, 33*(2), 362–377. doi: 10.5465/AMR.2008.31193235

Gittell, J. H. (2009). *High performance healthcare: Using the power of relationships to achieve quality, efficiency and resilience.* New York, NY: McGraw Hill Professional.

Hall, A., & Walton, G. (2004). Information overload within the health care system: A literature review. *Health Information & Libraries Journal, 21*(2), 102–108. doi: 10.1111/j.1471-1842.2004.00506.x

Heller, B. R., Drenkard, K., Esposito-Herr, M. B., Romano, C., Tom, S., & Valentine, N. (2004). Educating nurses for leadership roles. *Journal of Continuing Education in Nursing, 35*(5), 203.

Horton-Deutsch, S. (2013). Thinking it through: The path to reflective leadership. *American Nurse Today, 8*(2), 1–4.

Kanter, R. M. (2011). Zoom in, zoom out. *Harvard Business Review, 89*(3), 112–116.

Kellerman, B. (2012). *The end of leadership.* New York, NY: HarperCollins.

Kor, Y. Y., & Mesko, A. (2013). Dynamic managerial capabilities: Configuration and orchestration of top executives' capabilities and the firm's dominant logic. *Strategic Management Journal, 34*(2), 233–244. doi: 10.1002/smj.2000

Kotter, J. P. (2007). Leading change: Why transformation efforts fail. *Harvard Business Review, 85*(1), 96–103.

Kouzes, J. , & Posner, B. (2012). *The leadership challenge: How to make extraordinary things happen in organizations* (5th ed.). San Francisco, CA: Jossey-Bass.

Lichtenstein, B. B., & Plowman, D. A. (2009). The leadership of emergence: A complex systems leadership theory of emergence at successive organizational levels. *The Leadership Quarterly, 20*(4), 617–630.

Lichtenstein, B. B., Uhl-Bien, M., Marion, R., Seers, A., Orton, J. D., & Schreiber, C. (2006). Complexity leadership theory: An interactive perspective on leading in complex adaptive systems. *Emergence: Complexity & Organization, 8*(4), 2–12.

Lindberg, C., Nash, S., & Lindberg, C. (2008). *On the edge: Nursing in the age of complexity.* Bordentown, NJ: Plexus Press.

Lindberg, C., & Schneider, M. (2012). Leadership in a complex adaptive system: Insights from positive deviance. *Academy of Management Best Paper Proceedings, 2012.* Retrieved from http://www.plexusinstitute.org/?page=complexity10

Luthans, F. (2002). The need for and meaning of positive organizational behavior. *Journal of organizational behavior, 23*(6), 695–706.

McHugh, M. D., Kelly, L. A., Smith, H. L., Wu, E. S., Vanak, J. M., & Aiken, L. H. (2013). Lower mortality in magnet hospitals. *Medical Care, 51*(5), 382–388. doi: 10.1097/MLR.0b013e3182726cc5

Metcalf, L., & Benn, S. (2012). The corporation is ailing social technology: Creating a 'fit for purpose' design for sustainability. *Journal of Business Ethics, 111*(2), 195–210. doi: 10.1007/s10551-012-1201-1

Metcalf, L., & Benn, S. (2013). Leadership for sustainability: An evolution of leadership ability. *Journal of Business Ethics, 112*(3), 369–384. doi: 10.1007/s10551-012-1278-6

Northouse, P. (2013). *Leadership: Theory and practice* (6th ed.). Los Angeles, CA: Sage.

Oldroyd, J. B., & Morris, S. S. (2012). Catching falling stars: A human resource response to social capital's detrimental effect of information overload on star employees. *Academy of Management Review, 37*(3), 396–418.

Pink, D. H. (2011). *Drive: The surprising truth about what motivates us.* New York, NY: Penguin.

Porter-O'Grady, T. (2003). Nurses as knowledge workers. *Creative Nursing, 9,* 6.

Seiler, S., & Pfister, A. C. (2009). "Why did I do this?": Understanding leadership behavior through a dynamic five-factor model of leadership. *Journal of Leadership Studies, 3*(3), 41–52. doi: 10.1002/jls.20122

Stone, L. (2007). Living with continuous partial attention. *Harvard Business Review, 85*(2), 28.

Tan, J., Wen, H. J., & Awad, N. (2005). Health care and services delivery systems as complex adaptive systems. *Communications of the ACM, 48*(5), 36–44.

The American Nurses Credentialing Center. (2014). Magnet recognition program model. Retrieved from http://www.nursecredentialing.org/Magnet/NewMagnetModel.aspx#TransformationalLeadership

The Institute of Medicine at the National Academies. (2010). *The future of nursing: Focus on education.* Washington, D.C.: National Academy of Sciences. Retrieved from http://www.iom.edu/~/media/Files/Report%20Files/2010/The-Future-of-Nursing/Nursing%20Education%202010%20Brief.pdf

Tjan, A. (2012). How leaders become self-aware. Harvard Business Review Blog. Retrieved from http://blogs.hbr.org/2012/07/how-leaders-become-self-aware/

Uhl-Bien, M., Marion, R., & McKelvey, B. (2007). Complexity leadership theory: Shifting leadership from the industrial age to the knowledge era. *The Leadership Quarterly, 18*(4), 298–318.

Waltuck, Bruce A. (2012). Complexity and leadership. *Journal for Quality & Participation, 35*(1), 1–3.

Youssef, C. M., & Luthans, F. (2007). Positive organizational behavior in the workplace the impact of hope, optimism, and resilience. *Journal of Management, 33*(5), 774–800.

Zimmerman, B., Lindberg, C., & Plsek, P. (2001). *Edgeware: Insights from complexity science for health care leaders.* Irving, TX: VHA.

5

Clinical Nurse Specialists (CNSs) as Change Agents

Terri Bogue, MSN, RN, PCNS
and Robert L. Bogue, MCSE, CNA

"Whereas novices may be confused by all the data elements, experts see the big picture, and they appear to be less likely to fall victim to information overload."

—Sources of Power (Klein, 1998)

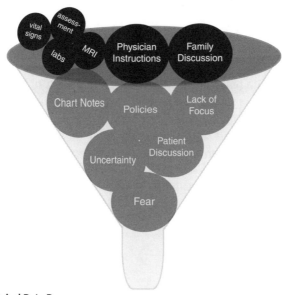

FIGURE 5. **Clinical Data Dump**

Information overload for the healthcare system has grown at epidemic proportions. Healthcare workers are bombarded by more tests, diagnostics, and information than at any time in history. As a result, there is more information to process, respond to, and decipher. Never in the history of human civilization have we had so much information to process on a daily basis. For instance, *The Paradox of Choice* (Schwartz, 2005) says that the average American sees 3,000 advertisements a day, while *Guerilla Marketing* (Levinson, 2007) says that we're bombarded by approximately 4,700 advertisements every day. While in the broader experience of humans it is disturbing and concerning, in health care information overload can have disastrous consequences.

However, information overload is more than just the quantity of facts and figures streaming in front of us. Information overload is more a statement about our ability as professionals to process the data that we have and to make sense of it without becoming overwhelmed by it. In fact, the role of the CNS is often to integrate additional information that the system doesn't normally have. This is done through research and finding evidence to improve patient outcomes, nurse effectiveness, and system outcomes and thinking. The CNS frequently acts as a change agent to improve the processing of information so that it does not lead to overload. The CNS has numerous competencies and skills that can be leveraged to this end (National CNS Competency Task Force, 2014). This chapter focuses on how to effect change through these competencies and skills.

The Information Problem

The starting point for any effort to resolve an information overload problem is to understand the problem itself. While healthcare workers face more information now than even a few short years ago, this is not the sole problem. The real problem is that as the rate of change in health care has increased, the entropy of the information that we do have has increased, and it is becoming more difficult for everyone to understand what the right answers are. It is more and more difficult to detect the signal amongst the noise when the signal keeps changing. The rate of change for the industry and the rate at which new evidence is created and discovered means that change is a very real part of the information overload challenge facing healthcare workers today.

The CNS Solution

The CNS addresses the challenges of information overload and the pace of change by working within three spheres of influence: the patient/family unit, the nurse, and the system. The CNS creates change constructed on evidence-based research for the purpose of creating better outcomes for the patient. These changes to support evidence-based research would seem to further negatively impact the information overload problem. However, when implemented correctly, these changes can reduce cognitive load and the complexity of task demands. However, when implemented correctly, these changes can improve clarity and reduce cognitive load as a result of reducing task complexity. In the example that follows, clarifying the standards for central-line care and providing productivity tools reduced the complexity of the task and decreased confusion, thereby reducing cognitive load. The lack of clarity, increased cognitive load, and unnecessary complexity of determining appropriate practices prevent well-intended nurses from delivering on their desire for the best care for their patients.

When individuals are confronted with a lack of clarity they tend not to take action (McChesney, Covey, & Huling, 2012). As a result, one of the key activities of a CNS during the process of change (described below) is to create clarity. The CNS must also ensure that the tools are available to communicate with the healthcare team and support their continued understanding. This process is directly related to the CNS core competencies: consultation, system leadership, collaboration, research, and coaching (National CNS Competency Task Force, 2014).

By incorporating evidence-based practice, the CNS creates clarity around what the optimal policy and practice should be. By using evidence and information selectively, and through inter-disciplinary collaboration, facilitating meetings, and leveraging their relationships with the entire care team, the CNS can develop a single, clear policy statement related to a specific practice that eliminates ambiguity and addresses the concerns of the healthcare workers. An example of incorporating evidence-based practice was evident as practice changes in nursing occurred related to turning patients in the ICU for pressure ulcer prevention. Previously there was a belief that patients' lives were being saved in the ICU, and that pressure ulcers would heal if the patients survived. Yet this did not always occur, and it became imperative that more focus should be placed on prevention of pressure ulcers during an ICU stay. The CNS's influence resulted in the evidence-based practice of utilization of the Braden Q Scale to predict pressure ulcers. This information relates to the prevention of pressure ulcers before they occur and definitive practice changes that have become a standard of practice. These changes are possible only through collaboration with the entire healthcare team and CNS leadership.

Using system leadership skills and approaches, the CNS can reduce the rate of change to a practice policy to only the essential. This reduces the amount of unnecessary information communicated to the staff. The CNS ensures that policy changes occur only when necessary. They reduce the number of changes to a policy by coordinating multiple changes into a single change packet that is processed as a unit. The CNS works to maintain stability and evidenced-based practice in the hospital system. This stability and attention to the frequency of change reduces information overload by removing unnecessary noise and confusion.

The CNS begins to manage information overload using evidence-based decisions for practice. This is followed by collaboration with educators and managers to develop a set of communication tools that are designed to clearly articulate what is expected of every staff member. Thus, the "why" for the practice is included whenever possible, and decisions are documented into a policy that will guide practice on the unit. These communication tools include the traditional instructor-led materials for the initial training as well as the productivity aids that are essential to minimizing the cognitive load—and therefore information overload—of the workers as they seek to execute the policy.

Finally, the CNS integrates into the execution of the policy and practice changes the feedback loop necessary to improve the educational materials and productivity aids. They also identify barriers preventing the successful execution of the policy. This critical feedback loop is necessary to ensure the reduction in information overload and that the advances gained are sustained in the system over the long term.

Case Study: Central Line-Associated Bloodstream Infections (CLABSI) Reductions

To better illustrate the role, the CNS should play a change agent. The following situation describes how frequently changing rules and excessive noise related to central line care caused significant information overload and substantial practice variation. This resulted in a non-trivial number of avoidable negative outcomes including preventable infections, longer hospital stays, and in some cases, may have been a contributing factor to patient mortality.

Sally begins her position after the unit has made multiple significant changes to their central line bundle. The changes in the bundle seem to come rapidly, and nurses are frustrated that they do not know what the appropriate steps of the bundle are. When she starts, CLABSI rates are at an all-time low of 1.3 per 1,000 line days. Within her first year, the rates double, and the bedside nurses caring for the patients, the managers, the chief nursing officer, and the hospital CEO are concerned. There is confusion, frustration, and a sense of cognitive overload that makes previous improvements impossible to maintain.

Sally, a new CNS, walks into this situation and soon recognizes that information overload is causing the increase in CLABSI rates. The real question Sally faces is how to develop a specific evidence-based bundle, change the beliefs around central line care, and reduce the detrimental effects of information overload.

Sally recognizes that as central lines become more necessary in practice, staff are caring for more and more patients with central lines. As these central lines are accessed more frequently, the patients seem sicker, causing new and more complicated medications to be administered through central lines, and more laboratory results and assessments that need to be interpreted.

Sally begins her assessment by observing the daily care of patients. She soon identifies the ever-increasing volumes of information from the increased diagnostic tests and assessments that the nurses process every hour. Sally begins to understand that the frequency of access and longevity of the lines has created a significant risk of central line infection.

Sally talks to the nurses about the current central line bundle. The nurses share that they are inundated with sometimes conflicting information related to the prevention of central line infections. They receive emails from different sources including the previous CNS, managers, line experts, and educators providing information related to care of central lines. Conflicting information in these messages leads to confusion about what to do next. Sally quickly realizes that it is difficult for the nurses to evaluate what the greatest risks to the patients truly are. In addition, the nurses share with Sally that the bundle and the procedures change almost monthly. This is further complicated by the nurses' friends on other units who hear something different and share their understanding of proper care. Sally soon realizes there is more to the increasing CLABSI rates than just the evidence-based bundle.

Complicating matters, the hospital leadership believes that the nurses are responsible for the increasing CLABSI rate. They share this belief with the nurses by telling them that they are responsible for the rate change and the resulting harm this causes the patients. This creates feelings of guilt and shame among the nurses that make it more difficult for them to perform effectively. Infection rates double on the unit that Sally supports, going from 1.3 CLABSI per 1,000 line days to 2.6 CLABSI per 1,000 line days in less than one year. The nurses feel personally responsible for the infections.

No one knows where to find a current printed version of the bundle, and they all know that the new bundle is not reflected in the current policy. There is much confusion and discussion related to what appropriate central line care really entails.

Sally realizes that the nurses personally feel responsible for harm to their patients, yet they also feel powerless to prevent it. The quantity of information and the lack of clarity create a great deal of anxiety and information overload for the nurses. They soon feel hopeless in being able to change the situation and their course of action is unclear. The nurses do not know what they need to do to be successful. More pressure to "do better" and to "be safer" doesn't help the nurses understand what specifically they should do to improve patient care.

To further complicate the problem, Sally soon discovers that the confusion among the nurses results in patients being treated differently by different nurses. The patients are being told different expectations for the care required of their central line. The patients are confused by the different practices and instructions. As a result, the patients lose trust and confidence in the nurses and their entire healthcare team. This further intensifies their fear of hospital-acquired infection. This loss of trust is significant as 82% of people list nursing as the most trusted profession (Gallop, Inc, 2013). The nurse holds this trust sacred and strives to continue to earn the patients' trust on a daily basis.

Based on her assessment of the scope and basis of the problem, Sally knows that she only has one chance to make all the changes required and provide a clear and standardized process not only for the units she is responsible for but for the entire population. The research, collaboration, system leadership, and coaching skills Sally has as a CNS will be tested to reduce information overload, standardize an evidence-based practice, and support a positive change.

Sally draws on her knowledge of the collaborative competency of the CNS to facilitate the healthcare team in engaging in patient-, family-, and system-focused problem solving to optimize clinical outcomes (National CNS Competency Task Force, 2014). Sally also provides indirect care to the patients through activities that influence the care provided to them through the development of evidence-based protocols for patient care and staff development (National CNS Competency Task Force, 2014).

Sally works with the hospital-acquired condition committee, which includes physicians, infection preventionists, and nurses, to approve the updated evidence-based bundle. Sally then updates the central line policy with the new guidelines developed in the updated bundle and works with the hospital policy and procedure committee to get the revised policy approved. Sally's next step is to collaborate with the education department to develop education of the new bundle and policy. She knows that "why it works" and "why it's important" are fundamental questions for nurses that help them discern what to do when their professional judgment is required to administer care that at times does not have a black and white answer. Once the nurses understand the rationale behind the bundle, it is much easier to determine when dressings need changing or what care is most appropriate to reduce the risk of infection. The education that is created

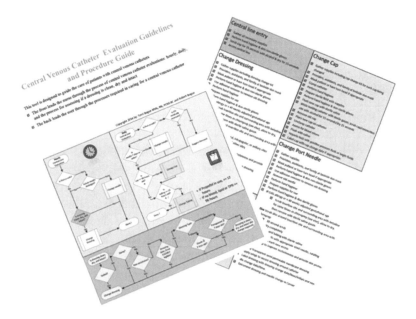

FIGURE 6. **Central Line Productivity Aid**

has time buildt in for the nurses to discuss concerns with the new practice and have the "why" further clarified. It places importance on the patient, family, and nurse rather than rates, allowing the nurses to correlate their desire to care for their patient with the real risk that a central line infection presents. This empowers the nurses to exercise professional judgment and reduced their feeling of helplessness.

At this point Sally knows that she is encountering success. She also knows that the process is not complete. She develops an auditing process that includes systematic feedback to the nurses. She collaborates with the unit managers to secure the necessary support to assure compliance. Next, Sally helps to implement an auditing process to assess which nurses are voluntarily implementing the new guidelines and which nurses need more encouragement to follow the updated policy and implement the updated bundle.

While the infections are dropping substantially, Sally takes each infection as an opportunity to learn how to do better. Working with the nurses, Sally looks for root causes for the infections. Even before the infections are confirmed, the nurses are identifying probable root causes themselves. This is when Sally knows that she has given nurses the ability to take better care of their patients.

Sally successfully implemented a new policy in such a way that the confusion that caused information overload was significantly reduced. She will continue to follow the same process when implementing change in the future. This leads to many successful implementations of evidence-based change and a reduction in information overload for staff.

CNS as Change Agent

In this case, the CNS was the change agent who supported and helped the nurses to believe and reduce the number of CLABSI in their patients. The nurses gained the knowledge, support, and tools to provide the required care without confusion or conflict. Their success rates improved, their information overload was decreased, and their patients' outcomes improved. The patients' trust and confidence in their nurses increased as they could see the confidence the nurses had in their knowledge and abilities. The hospital appreciated the change in CLABSI rates, patient satisfaction, and effects of the reduction in information overload for their staff. The CNS clearly impacted all three spheres of influence to improve outcomes on several levels. Each sphere provided improvement for the next in a flow that resulted in consistently reduced information overload (Figure 7).

As the CNS works to incorporate change in the three spheres of influence, ultimately, they're attempting to bring into harmony the communications that each receives and sends to the other spheres. The process is about simplifying messages to reduce information overload and create clarity.

The Process of Clarity

The case study above demonstrates the capacity of the CNS to develop a clarity that reduces the amount and severity of the impact of information overload on nurses and patients. The process of clarity, developed by the authors, provides a structured framework for the development of clarity in a healthcare environment. In this section, we will demonstrate how this process of clarity works, and provide specific recommendations for how to generate the clarity necessary to dispel information overload.

Define the Standard

When there is a lack of a defined standard of care or accepted professional practice, and the current policy does not match the perceived standard of care, a great deal of time and effort is spent with different parties arguing over the areas where there is a lack of alignment. We have all been a part of meetings that get lost in some unimportant aspect of a policy that no one cares about.

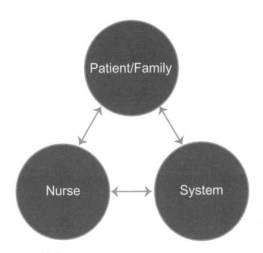

FIGURE 7. **CNS spheres of influence**

Standards of care in this context are the agreements about how things are expected to be completed. These standards of care should match policy, yet frequently are changed without policy being updated. They may also reflect practice that does not have a related policy. This could be recorded in a formal written standard of care or could be a unit-based standard that is recognized but not documented anywhere. These issues lead to unnecessary work complexity and ineffective policies. The process of defining the standard of care and evolving it to clarity is the process of developing a single, unarguable standard of care and effective policy that will reduce the amount of energy spent arguing about differences of opinions. This process decreases cognitive burden and unnecessary work complexity that lead to information overload.

The process for defining the standard is as follows:

1. **Identify the specific goal**—What was the root cause of the problem(s) and what specific intervention(s) do you believe can make a difference? In the case study above, it was reducing the information overload related to the care of central lines.

2. **Gather the stakeholders**—Identify all of the parties who need to be represented in finding a solution and agreeing to standards of care. In the case study above, there were the doctors, nurses, infection prevention, and administration (since they would be purchasing supplies).

3. **Gather relevant evidence**—The role of the CNS is, in part, to bring evidence-based practice to the organization. This process of gathering the relevant research and including it as a part of the discussion for improving the solution is critical to minimizing the number of disagreements and to the formation of a shared opinion.

4. **Create an environment for consensus and agreement**—The CNS creates a forum for dialogue that allows each party's concerns and perspectives to be brought together where consensus can be reached.

5. **Create buy-in**—While consensus is good, creating real buy-in, where all of the parties will defend the group decision, is key to ensuring that variations of the message don't create the same information overload problem with which we started. Buy-in itself is getting the key stakeholders to confirm and commit to the consensus, and often involves a few more people to test that the resulting decision is coherent and clear.

Education and Performance Support

Education is the up-front push to get everyone on to the new standard. Performance support is the supporting infrastructure that helps to ensure that the training is retained and that the new standard is followed. Education is the burst of energy to break the inertia of the status quo. Kotter, for instance, proposes an eight-step change model, the first step of which is creating a sense of urgency (Kotter & Cohen, 2012). Performance support is the sustaining energy that keeps things moving forward. All too often education isn't supported and eventually behavior regresses to the point it was before the education. Performance support is necessary to anchor education in the hearts and minds of the organization.

Education

In general, interactive learning experiences such as those provided by on-the-job mentoring and coaching are the most impactful because the training is done in the context of how it will be used. However, this is often prohibitively expensive because the scale is one instructor teaching one, or perhaps two, provider(s) at a time. Instructor-led training in a classroom setting still allows for interaction without the benefit of same-context. The benefit, however, of instructor-led training is that it offers better leverage in a classroom setting and can therefore be more cost-effective.

Solutions with computer-based training are, generally speaking, much more difficult and time-consuming to develop—particularly when using techniques like quizzes and non-video elements. The lack of ability to ask questions means that the effectiveness of the learning is reduced. However, computer-based training does have the advantage of lower costs in comparison to on-the-job or instructor-led training. Dead last on the list of effective training options are printed materials because there's no way to truly ensure that people will actually work through the materials. They're very scalable, but they're also ineffective.

The following flow chart demonstrates how focusing on the salient factors can take a complex decision and reduce the cognitive load. By answering only three key questions about a situation it is possible to reach a clear decision about what kind of education to create. The decision related to the type of education developed should be based on the following factors as shown in Figure 8:

1. **How many practitioners do you need to initially train?**—If the standard impacts only a small number of people it may be possible to do on-the-job mentoring and coaching, but in most cases you'll need to look at a solution that's much more scalable.

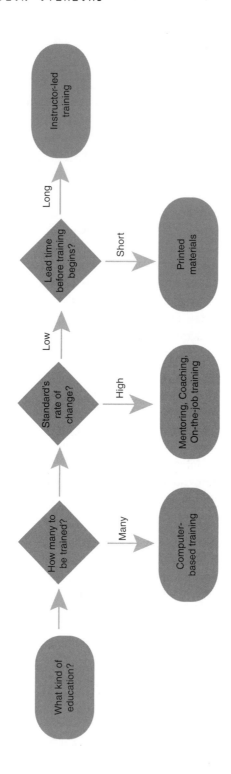

FIGURE 8. **Simplified Educational Approach Decision**

2. **How stable do you expect the standard to be?**—If the standard tracks governmental regulations that change infrequently, then the time and energy to develop a computer-based training solution may be appropriate—this is particularly true if training for compliance to the standard that you've developed must be reportable. Conversely, if you're leaving flexibility to change the standard next quarter, developing computer-based training isn't the best choice.

3. **How much time do you have before you train?**—If you need to resolve the issue immediately and reach compliance with the standard you've developed, it may require on-the-job solutions that require relatively little preparation. Instructor-led materials can generally be developed quickly if necessary, whereas computer-based training solutions have a much longer lead time for development.

Productivity Aids

Productivity aids are one particularly effective method of performance support. They are tools that aid in professional decision making as well as act as a reminder for specific actions that must be taken. Where education happens one time, productivity aids can be accessed over and over again to ensure that the behavior matches the standard.

The checklist is a productivity aid that was designed specifically to deal with the information overload problem. Atul Gawande speaks about the Boeing Model 299, which crashed during a test flight due to the test pilot being unable to manage the complexity of the aircraft. The solution to the unmanageable complexity was a humble checklist that reduced reliance on memory. The craft ultimately became the venerable B-17 bomber with over 1.8 million miles with the help of a checklist (Gawande, 2009).

Checklists aren't the only type of productivity aid available. Another popular productivity aid is a flow chart or decision tree. A flow chart or decision tree can help focus practitioners on the most important and critical decisions, and the order in which they should be made. By referring to other processes or standards, even complex processes can be represented in ways that allow practitioners to make decisions quickly. By focusing practitioners on critical information they are necessarily assisted in filtering unnecessary and distracting information.

When developing decision trees, it's often difficult to articulate the specific criteria; however, this is specifically why decision trees are valuable. By distilling the general guidance into the specific criteria it becomes possible to get consistent results. For instance, in the case study above the challenge was how to assess whether the dressing needed to be changed. Ultimately the statement "clean, dry, and intact" became the set of criteria for dressing changes. These words were clear enough to be well understood by all the nurses and were simple enough to represent in a diamond (decision point) on the decision tree.

In the case study, the productivity aid that was developed used both a flow chart and a checklist to ensure consistent behaviors from all of the nurses.

Performance

The implementation of a productivity aid is done around areas where performance can or must be improved. Here are some criteria for implementing productivity aids:

1. Is this a place where compliance to the standard of practice is inconsistent? Though not often well known at the beginning of the process, informed guesses can be made about areas of the standard which will be difficult to maintain. These are the key areas to support with productivity aids.

2. Is there a series of steps that must be completed in the same order for the same length of time whenever the procedure is performed? If so, then a checklist may help to ensure that the same steps are executed every time.

3. Is there a complex decision that may seem subjective but for which clear criteria can be developed? If you have what appear on the surface to be completely subjective decisions, the development of a decision tree can help you create clear rules to create consistent behaviors.

Accessibility

Even well-developed productivity aids will be useless if they're not well known to the people that need them and available at the time they need them. Solving the problem of accessibility of a productivity aid may be as simple as publishing the productivity aid to the intranet or knowledge repository. However, it may mean the printing and disbursement of the productivity aid to the unit, or even to the patients' rooms, so that it's available when it's needed most.

Compliance and Reinforcement

Mason Haire famously said, "What gets measured gets done" (Peters & Waterman, 1982). Even the best education and the most compelling productivity aids won't work if they're not supported by techniques to ensure compliance with the standard and efforts by the organization to reinforce the implementation of the standard.

Ensuring compliance with the standard is more than simply measuring the desired outcome. It's about measuring the behaviors called for in the standard. It's about auditing, checking, and verifying that what should be happening is actually happening. Here are three keys to compliance and reinforcement:

1. **Audit the behavior to the standard**—Verify that the behaviors called for by the standard are happening through random sampling.
2. **Report the results**—Report the results of the auditing and communicate them in an easy-to-understand form, such as a line chart showing the progress of compliance over time.
3. **Relate the results**—Relate the results of the audited behavior with the downstream intended impacts. As compliance with the standard is increased, the desired outcome is increased. It's expected that there will be variability in both metrics, but they should show a clear relationship.

Ensuring compliance to the standard reduces information overload by reducing the amount of cognitive capacity that must be used to assess the validity of the standard. By communicating clearly what the standard is, and—more importantly—that it's to be adhered to, cognitive load is decreased.

Continuous Improvement and Change Control

Having implemented the new standard isn't the end. The process described above in the case study continues today. There is new research that leads to opportunities to improve the standard. There are new changes in the environment that require small changes to the standard, as well. The role of the CNS to reduce information overload shifts from the simplification of the solution and creating clarity to a process that balances the need to take advantage of the latest evidence and to ensure that changes aren't happening so fast that they are creating the conditions for information overload.

The key questions before changing the standard are:

1. Are there changes to the environment or to research that would lead us to believe that there is a non-trivial gain that can be made by changing the process?
2. Would the gain in changing the process warrant the cost of the retraining and potential information overload?

Ultimately, the goal for updating standards is to remain flexible enough to take advantage of new opportunities while remaining rigid enough to avoid constant change.

Barriers to Success

Even with the best procedure for creating clarity, barriers will arise. These barriers can derail the process of creating clarity. They impede the process by impacting each of the participants in a personal and profound way. The three key barriers are: narrow focus due to stress, blame created from shame, and low trust from disengagement.

Stress Creates Narrow Focus

Imagine that you're presented with the task to affix a candle to the wall in a way that the wax doesn't drip onto a table. You're given a box of tacks, some matches, and a candle. Most people will stumble upon the solution of putting the candle on the box of tacks and using the tacks to affix the box to the wall. What's interesting is that people who are subjected to even a slight amount of stress, in the form of a financial reward for doing it quickly, will do worse. Functional fixedness, which prevents someone from thinking of the box holding the tacks as a part of the solution, is just one way that stress limits thinking (Pink, 2010).

As the cognitive load increases as more details and information accumulate, the nurse finds that their ability to assess the entire situation decreases due to stress. For example, a nurse enters a patient's room and finds the patient breathing rapidly, the monitor showing they are tachycardic with oxygen saturations in the mid 90s. The nurse immediately focuses on potential physical causes for the problem. Due to the stress of determining the cause of the problem, combined with the knowledge that there are other patients waiting for help, medications that are due, and IV pumps alarming, the nurse's focus is directed solely at the physical state of the patient. They may not notice that the patient's sibling had just told the patient something that caused them great anxiety. The nurse's focus is on quickly finding a solution for the patient's tachycardia and tachypnea: functional fixedness prevented the nurse from recognizing another potential cause of the problem.

Gary Klein specifically addresses the impact of stress on decision-making and concludes that

- Stressors do not give us a chance to gather as much information as possible
- Stressors disrupt our ability to use our working memory to sort things out
- Stressors distract our attention from the task at hand (Klein, 1998)

The main effect of stress on nurses, according to Paul Tough, is that "it compromises their ability to regulate their thoughts" (Tough, 2012). *Emotional Intelligence* catalogs numerous impacts of stress, including the physical effects (Goleman, 2006). Stress disrupts our ability to process the information we do get. It makes information overload easier, and as a result, our brains shut down the ability to process information; instead, we focus on a very narrow band of things that we already know and that are right in front of us. From an evolutionary standpoint, stress was designed to focus us during a time of eminent, personal danger. We, unlike zebras, can feel the effects of stress for non-life-threatening situations and for long periods of time (Sapolsky, 2004).

Some level of stress is inherent to our jobs, and ultimately becomes a part of the operating conditions, so it no longer affects us. However, a different kind of stress is created by uncertainty in the sustainability of our organizations and our departments. This stress is distracting to us and prevents us from doing our best work. Where possible, unnecessary and abnormal stressors should be removed from organizations to improve responses and reduce the impact of information overload.

Blame Creates Shame

In an era of increased accountability it's often hard to avoid a tendency to play the blame game because, as Brené Brown says, "Blame is simply the discharging of pain and discomfort" (Brown, 2012). That is the discomfort of our part in the problem. The key problem in playing the blame game is that it is often converted into guilt or shame on the part of the recipient. Guilt is the belief that you did something bad. Shame is the belief that you *are* bad. Shame is a debilitating feeling. In her research, Dr. Brown describes shame as the secret killer of innovation. Shame is a deep fear that you cannot be good, and fear is the primary creator of stress—the very thing that limits our ability to function.

Low Trust Creates Disengagement

At one level, trust is painfully simple to create. You need only to make a commitment and meet the commitment—or renegotiate the commitment before it's due. On the other hand, trust is widely misunderstood. You may trust your babysitter to watch your children. You may trust your accountant to do your taxes. However, would you trust your babysitter to do your taxes or your accountant to watch your children? Trust is relationship- and context-based.

With all the confusion around what trust is, it's little wonder that organizations suffer from a crisis of trust. Trust is eroded by the small commitments that are missed, whether it's the implicit commitment to be treated with respect as a professional or the commitment to communicate clearly and directly.

The impact of a low level of trust is seen as disengagement by the organization. However, the path to disengagement has many stops. Employees that don't trust their organization (or manager) believe that anything is possible—even scary things. This leads to fear and stress which focus them back on only those things that are essential to their survival, and thus they're unable to come up with creative contributions to move the organization forward.

Tools and Tips

Table 4 briefly summarizes the tools and techniques that the CNS can use to reduce the impact of information overload.

Summary

Information overload is a challenge that we all face in our daily lives and in our professional work. We're bombarded by too much information and have too little time to react. By supporting the development of clear messages the CNS can dramatically reduce the impact of information overload on nurses, patients, and the system.

Sometimes the tools for creating clarity are both simple and seldom used. For instance, throughout this chapter we've highlighted key points in bulleted and numbered lists to create a focusing effect to reduce the impact of information overload even from this chapter.

A final note on the CNS as a change agent: The best CNS acknowledges that they are not able to be a change agent alone. They have mentors and supporters that allow them to do things they never believed possible.

TABLE 4. **Tools and Techniques to Reduce Impact of Information Overload**

Key Idea	Rationale and Implementation
Identify appropriate stakeholders	In health care, there are many stakeholders who care for a patient. Start by identifying the parties who need to be involved. Use project management tools like RACI charts to clarify what role each stakeholder plays.
Assess clarity	Testing proposed changes with the nurses who have to implement them can help to expose any places where the intended meaning might not be clear. Consider games which encourage nurses to compete for bragging rights about finding the most important oversight of the changes.
Consistency is Key	Any time that messages aren't consistent between parties or that policies and procedures don't match, a substantial amount of confusion will be created. Encourage staff to raise issues of consistency and create a process for resolving them.
Teach the Why and the How	Education is frequently focused on the "how" and not the "why." In cases where professional judgment is required, like where there are competing factors for risk, it's necessary to teach "why" as well. Consider adding scenarios to your education for which there is no right answer but that will elicit the discussion on important factors.
Create Productivity Aids	Checklists and flow charts are seemingly small, however, their ability to continuously reinforce standards and processes are impressive. Create checklists when possible. See The Checklist Manifesto for more on the impact of checklists (Gawande, 2009).
Information Access	Information that can't be accessed can't be used. Place policies and procedures in places that are physically or electronically easy for the staff to access quickly. Productivity aids should be made available in physical form where possible.
Audit Compliance	Overcoming the initial resistance to change requires monitoring. Establish simple approaches for ensuring that the new behaviors are becoming habits.
Create Feedback Loops	Reinforce the good news that the expected outcome is moving in the right direction, and create opportunities for root cause analysis when an occurrence is moving away from the desired outcome.

References

Brown, B. (2012). *Daring greatly*. New York: Gotham Books.

Gallop, Inc. (2013). *Honesty/ethics in professions*. Retrieved from http://www.gallup.com/poll/1654/Honesty-Ethics-Professions.aspx

Gawande, A. (2009). *The checklist manifesto*. New York, NY: Metropolitan Books.

Goleman, D. (2006). *Emotional intelligence: 10th anniversary edition*. New York, NY: Bantam Dell.

Klein, G. (1998). *Sources of power: How people make decisions*. Cambridge, MA: MIT Press.

Kotter, J., & Cohen, D. (2012). *The heart of change*. Boston, MA: Harvard Business Review Press.

Levinson, J. (2007). *Guerrilla marketing: Easy and inexpensive strategies for making big profits from your small business* (4th ed.). Boston, MA: Houghton Mifflin.

McChesney, C., Covey, S., & Huling, J. (2012). *The 4 disciplines of execution*. New York, NY: Simon and Schuster.

Nader, R. (1965). *Unsafe at any speed: The designed-in dangers of the American automobile*. New York, NY: Grossman.

National CNS Competency Task Force. (2014). *Clinical nurse specialst core competencies*. Harrisburg, PA: National Association of Clinical Nurse Speicalist.

Peters, T., & Waterman, R. (1982). *In search of excellence: Lessons from America's best-run companies*. New York, NY: Harper & Row.

Pink, D. (2010). Drive: *The surprising truth about what motivates us*. New York, NY: Riverhead Books.

Sapolsky, R. (2004). *Why zebras don't get ulcers*. New York, NY: Macmillan.

Schwartz, B. (2005). *The paradox of choice: Why more is less*. New York, NY: HarperCollins.

Tough, P. (2012). *How children succeed: Grit, curiosity, and the hidden power of character*. New York, NY: Houghton Mifflin Harcourt.

6

Supporting Leaders Through Complexity and Information Overload: Interview with a Nurse Executive Leader

Linda Q. Everett, PhD, RN, FAAN

Interview by
Marion E. Broome, PhD, RN, FAAN

Dr. Linda Q. Everett is currently Executive Vice President and Chief Nurse Executive of Indiana University Health and Associate Dean for Clinical Affairs of Indiana University School of Nursing. She has spent the last three decades in nursing leadership positions, all within academic medical centers. Dr. Everett has served as President of the Association of Nursing Executives (AONE) and chaired the AACN-AONE Task Force developing guidelines for Academic–Practice Partnerships. She has published widely about the complexity of the practice environment. In this interview, Dr. Everett, an experienced healthcare system nurse executive, shares her reflections and wisdom to reveal how leadership is an emotional state grounded in core values, and how leadership competencies are essential to lead and manage in a volatile, uncertain, chaotic, and ambiguous world.

MEB   Health care is restless right now. So how does an individual lead in a volatile, uncertain, and chaotic time in health care? What are the core values one must hold on to?

LQE   We just had our NEC summer retreat and the theme of that retreat was reflection and renewal and reflecting back on our best selves as a group. Part of the pre-reading assignment was an article by Robert Quinn (2005). Dr. Quinn talks about a fundamental state of leadership. Four points he brings out in his work were relevant to this question of leading in uncertain times. Quinn states that stressful times/chaotic times/times of uncertainty and ambiguity bring out different behaviors in leaders. These leaders on a normal day just exhibit their normal leadership style. Then when there is some type of crisis, they kick into a different level of behavior he calls "a fundamental state of leadership." In that article he does a nice job for me of segmenting in and outlining how I deal with uncertainty and chaos in an organization.

MEB   Can you describe that for me?

LQE   Quinn talks about leadership as an emotional state. You have your comfort centers—you're in your comfort zone—even as a leader, you have your comfort zone in a normal state and you stick with what you know. But in a uncertain/turbulent period of time, you go beyond that—you go beyond the comfort zone, you pursue other ambitious and new outcomes to solve the problem, whatever it is, so you move from a comfort zone to a non-comfort zone. For instance, in a normal period of time you're externally directed and comply with others' wishes in an effort to keep the peace ... okay ... so you compromise more. But when the chips are down and you're in a bind, you begin to behave in line with your own values so you become internally directed. You move from being externally directed to internally directed, falling back on your core values. The third state he talks about is one in which one becomes self-focused ... in normal times, you place your own interests above those of the group. However, in a difficult time, you put the collective good first. What's good for the whole, not what is good for me. Then the last principle is related to how and when one becomes internally closed. In normal times, you block out external stimuli in order to stay on task and avoid risk, but in these turbulent times, you learn from the environment and you recognize when there is a need for change.

So, really I think his conceptualization of the fundamental state of leadership is a really good way of describing how I deal with the chaos in this work environment. His paper, in the Harvard Business Review, is just really packed full of some real common sense—it's not necessarily a scholarly article, but it does really put this health-care environment into a context that I can relate to.

MEB What is interesting about those four points is that it seems like for some people those would seem like contradictory states. But good leaders in a crisis learn to manage those contradictions of emotion. For instance, looking inward to self when things are stable, but looking outwards toward others in the organization when times are turbulent, so to make the best decisions for the organization.

LQE You asked also about what are the core values that I have lived by during my entire career. Well, I went into nursing because I wanted to work with people and I wanted to help people, and at that time, those people became patients for me. I've always really tried to—in whatever situation that I've been in, whether that of a direct care provider and then a supervisor and so on up in the hierarchy—I really do try to think what's best for our patients and their families. As I got older, my family members became patients, you know, and I extended that fundamental core value to what is best for them. So that really guided my career, and I've always really tried to build upon that and enhance that by continuous learning. You know, I was a diploma nurse and went back and got a BSN, got a master's, got a doctorate, went to the Wharton program, and continually stay engaged with my organizations. I also stay engaged in professional associations so that I can just really refine my perspective and my intentions around trying to do the best that we can for taking care of patients—whatever that is in whatever setting. So that (i.e., continuous learning and development) just really has been a core value of mine. I believe when patients come to us, whether they come to us in an acute care setting, an ambulatory setting or home care, or offices or whatever, they're vulnerable. They're at risk and they're relying on nurses, physicians, and others ... but you know they really are placing their lives in a significant way in our care, and I take that very seriously.

MEB So, in light of all of that, how do you select leaders? Who you think will align with those core values? Who also help you to lead in these times? What kind of attributes do you look for?

LQE Well, #1 of course is that they have to be competent ... demonstrate a competency in nursing at some level. I wouldn't drill it down to a certain clinical level, but they have to be competent nurses in good standing within the profession ... that goes without saying, that that is the number one criterion. Someone shared with me one time when we were doing job interviews for a particular position that they interviewed several people for a high level executive job and that several of the candidates were really nice, but one had really a better handle on the work and, you know, seemed to express a higher level of competency. That individual asked my opinion, and I said, "you know what? I know a lot of nice people in this organization; I know a really select few of people that I would say are highly competent and could really do the job well." So, I really do put a lot of value on demonstrating that you know what the work is, whatever that work may be. If it's leading an operating room or it's leading one of the hospitals as a CNO, you obviously have to demonstrate in an interview or in your work that you can not only have critical thinking skills and clinical reasoning abilities, whatever you want to call it, but a leader must also have the ability to look at complex problems and be able to identify a solution. So I think being able to do that—be able to analyze the complexity of a problem and then take action on it—is critical.

When I look for leaders, I use behavioral interviewing techniques and give them scenarios and say, "How would you handle this?" I look for that process—their assessment of the complexity of the problem—and ask "were you able to identify the key pieces. Were you able to put it in a context where you could analyze it and then have an action plan on how to address it?" Now it might not be the right action plan, but at least they can verbalize what they would do about it.

I look for that, and I also look for personality and goodness of fit of a leader. Every organization has its own culture ... every unit ... every nursing unit, every work unit, wherever it is—the way people behave, the values that they collectively ascribe to, those types of things—they are all different and you have to, when you're selecting a leader to lead that group, you really need to have someone who can integrate with the group. And if the culture is not a positive one, will that person have the ability to change that culture over time? So it's not only a goodness of fit for what is, but does that person have the ability to move those they work with to a different level? Whether it be service-oriented, patient-care-oriented, financially-oriented, or whatever it is, the culture might not be a healthy one, but the individual is going to have to be able to in some way identify with it and then decide if it's a healthy culture. And if it's not a healthy culture, ask themselves how do I move it? So I look for those types of characteristics in leaders and of course the other things that you look for when you're choosing somebody just like when you're choosing faculty—you look at their track record ... where have they been, what have they done, how often have they moved, are they a job-hopper—what do they do? Are they spoiled? Engaged? Committed? Those types of things ...

MEB So that's a great segue in to this next question—so if a young nurse manager is interested in taking a culture or unit to the next level, how would you advise them to develop those skills? I know younger emerging leaders who have confidence to lead in the area they are currently in. But then, when in a new role or challenging area, they worry a bit about "how do I take something to the next level? How do I know what the next level is?" What would your recommendations be for them?

LQE   I think the first thing a young nurse manager needs to do is to have a mentor ... some people call them coaches, I call them mentors. Identify a mentor, someone who is a more seasoned person who can help guide and coach and work with the individual to help them identify those components within the culture, within the context, within the environment, that are positive and those things that aren't positive. Then talk over with this person: what are the challenges? How would you resolve them? Give the new manager options to choose from those types of activities. But again I go back to this whole thing about life-long learning and continuous development. I know at IU Health, and I think certainly most academic centers, have continuous learning development programs that staff and leaders can access if they are willing to do so. Now, they have to take initiative to do that. I would tell them, "Somebody's not going to come knock on your door and say here—I have this great class I want you to go to." Your coach or mentor might do that, but the individual has to be self-directed to do that, by pulling on resources. You know, don't be isolated, reach out, tap in to your network, develop a network. I'm where I am today because early in my career I started to develop a professional network of other leaders that didn't necessarily think the way I did, but they were leaders in their own right in other environments, and I would tap in to them, just like you do with listservs and other resources like that. In my experience, what many managers don't do enough of is reaching out beyond their unit, beyond their organization, beyond their hospital, to the greater world out there. They don't ask, "What is the best practice?" or "How can I improve upon this?" I think it's just recognizing that they don't have all the answers, and we don't expect them to have all the answers!

MEB   Right—benchmarking and looking around is a good idea.

LQE   Now, I don't expect them to be perfect. A lot of times, even today, we pluck a good staff nurse out of the ranks because we're desperate, because we don't have anybody to fill in—and you throw them into these jobs and then sometimes you're disappointed and dismayed that they weren't successful. That's like pushing a baby bird out of the nest when the poor thing hasn't flown ... and so we realize that, and we're trying to take steps in the acute care environment to correct that ... but again, it's changing that whole culture and the mindset of senior leaders ... about that. You're setting people up to fail when you don't give them the proper tools.

MEB And that leads into the next question—what is your recommendation about what they should do to develop emerging leaders? What kind of other opportunities and challenges should they get if they're assigned a mentor or assigned as a mentor? What should seasoned leaders provide the emerging leader with and how would they know that that person has actually grown and taken the opportunity?

LQE Well, there are a number of programs now internal to this organization, as well as external opportunities. American Organization of Nurse Executives (AONE) has a program, the Voluntary Hospital Association group has a program … and there are some other more expensive programs for aspiring nurse leaders. I believe investing in those individuals is a wise thing for the organization to do … getting them excited about learning and signing them up for these programs. We have sent three brand-new nurse managers from one of our hospitals to the AONE Emerging Leader Fellowship—it's a year-long fellowship. And that cost us money to do that, but we're investing in these people in the short-run to get long-term gain. University Hospital is going to send some people there as well … we have to dig around and find foundation monies to do this because taking it from operations right now is not something that would go over really well, but we're looking to develop them. How do you ensure they are taking advantage of such opportunities and growing? Well, if you're sending them to an external program— sometimes that's easier, because you know whether they went or not—and when they come back, we sit down and do de-briefs with them. We ask: What did you learn? How did you learn that? How would you apply that here? What exercises did you do in your two-day or week-long experience? That is, we ask them to tell us what they learned and how to apply it and then give them a project to do. You've got to keep them connected, you've got to keep them engaged … this isn't just a read one, do one, see one thing and then you put it on the shelf. You have to really use the tools you just learned about and apply them.

We have such a robust professional practice steering group here in each of the hospitals and each of the units has representatives to their hospital-based professional practice council and then to the system wide council, so we have them come here and share their stories. So, there is an accountability on the part of the participant as well as the immediate supervisor, the CNO in the facility, to see that people are not only taking advantage of the opportunities, but they come back and they apply it and then identify what are the outcomes of their growth as a leader.

MEB That is a good example of how to grow young leaders in an organization.

LQE Because a lot of times you see too—you see a lot of process—you see a lot of process in programs and you can't have outcomes unless you have structure and process, obviously. The ultimate questions are: did you improve the clinical outcomes of your patients? Did you address the financial effectiveness of your unit? Did you reduce the turnover of your staff nurses? Did you increase the teamwork and camaraderie of your unit? Tell me—what are your metrics and what did you do? And this is another thing I think that nurses struggle with—nurse managers and new managers in particular—are these metrics, and how do you know you made a difference if you don't measure it?

MEB   Is there anything that you think we have not talked about related to development of young leaders who must learn to lead in complex, dynamic environments of the future?

LQE   Well, I would just emphasize that these guidelines aren't for everyone. Again, you can be a great direct-care nurse, you can be a great CNS, but if we're talking about operational leadership, functional leadership in terms of running a unit or a department, or something like that, it takes a certain mindset or certain collection of skills that will enable you to again move from what is a normal state of leadership into these heightened turbulent crisis-type things. Just to give you an example, last winter, due to the looming fiscal challenges, we laid people off in this organization as our census dropped all through '13. Well, over the last several weeks, the census at all three of the larger hospitals was so high—so the question becomes: What do you do now? What if you don't have staff to take care of these people? We're going to have to close the operating rooms because we're running up against working the nurses over there up to the 60 hour rule—we can't work them over 60 hours ... It's not good for them and it's certainly not good for patients. So someone had to make the hard decision; senior leadership made the call last night: We have to close these operating rooms. Closing an operating room—that's like cutting off a water source—you might as well go home. But anyway, my point with that is—what are the options here? Now, if I go through those four points that I read from the Quinn article, you know, I think we went through every one of those at 7pm last night—patients are first here if you don't have qualified, competent, OR nurses to assist in those procedures, you're doing a disservice to that patient to bring that patient in ... so ... I had to elevate myself from my comfort zone. That was not a popular decision! It takes courage—that's another thing—it takes courage to be a leader—particularly when things are the way they are today and you have to really be able to stand by your beliefs.

MEB   And how could you justify that if something did go wrong?

LQE   So, you have to work out of your comfort zone, you have to step out of that and you have to say, "This is what I believe." I am willing to tell anyone "I'm the Chief Nurse here, if you don't want to take my advice, then you go out there and make that decision and you're going to be accountable for that decision." Of course I didn't have to go there, but the point of this is, not everybody can do that ... make that kind of decision.

MEB   It must be hard to step outside of the comfort zone and make unpopular decisions.

LQE   Right, it is. You have to have the facts, and you have to know what to do to resolve the problem. Sometimes it is really frustrating because an obvious solution to the problem is a system solution and workforce management. In this case though they wouldn't let us bring staff in from the outside surgery centers or from our other hospitals' operating room nurses that could come in and help because it's a different job code! Once I found that out, I said that until we figure this out we cannot operate. But just now I had a call right before this interview and I'm going to have another one when we're done here. I brought the HR people together and said, "We need a code—what do you have to do to get the right code so we can mobilize people and solve this problem?"

MEB   It sometimes seems this kind of scenario is pretty typical in any organization—if you had just caved and said well, you know, let's just do the unsafe care, one has to wonder what would happen. The organization has to choose: lose money or sacrifice patient care! That's amazing, and I'm sure that's true in any complex organization. A small barrier like the wrong job code can just absolutely throw everything into chaos.

LQE   So, to have somebody sit in a leader role that has the competence and courage to make a hard decision and believes that what they are doing is right for those patients, whether it's an operating room patient or it's a patient in ICU or labor and delivery and be able to stand by that when the slings and arrows start coming—that's tough—that's tough.

MEB   But I think the beautiful thing about this example is that if the code issue can be fixed, it's actually going a long way to address a larger issue which is how to deal with all of these fluctuations and staffing needs over time. It seems you're really looking at a basic systems problem—yeah, it's difficult right now, but if you can get that fixed as a result of this crisis ... that's going to enable you to deal with future crises.

LQE   It's a bureaucratic nightmare! Health care has entangled themselves into so many rules and regulations and you know what—we did it to ourselves. It's how you interpret the rules and regulations, and the joint commission will tell you that. Accreditors will give you a standard and then you get the organization's legal people and the risk people and all these other people who don't have to deliver care or document the care and then the rules tie you up in all of this red tape ... it's how we do that to ourselves.

MEB But to come back to your very first answer about core values. If you are patient-centered ... then you ... that's your first go-to. It's the big picture kind of thing ... and if the core value is always not following the bureaucratic rules, but following the rules for patient safety, then it's a whole different frame for decision-making. That's why I've always thought leaders with a clinician background have to be somewhere in the organization so they can reinforce the core value about patient safety.

Now, to wrap up: Do you think we have left anything unsaid in terms of how leaders shape and are shaped in our health care organizations?

LQE No, I think that says it all. Thanks for the opportunity to share my thoughts and experiences.

References

Quinn, R. (2003). *Moments of greatness: Entering the fundamental state of leadership.* Harvard Business Review, July 2005.

Index